SWINE DISEASE MANUAL

Fourth Edition

Edited by:
E.J. Neumann, A. Ramirez, and K.J. Schwartz

ISBN 978-0-9843503-0-8

Send orders to:

American Association of Swine Veterinarians
830 26th Street
Perry, Iowa 50220
Phone: 515-465-5255
Fax: 515-465-3832
E-mail: aasv@aasv.org
Order online: www.aasv.org/aasv/publications.htm

Formatting and cover design
Tina Smith

About The Cover

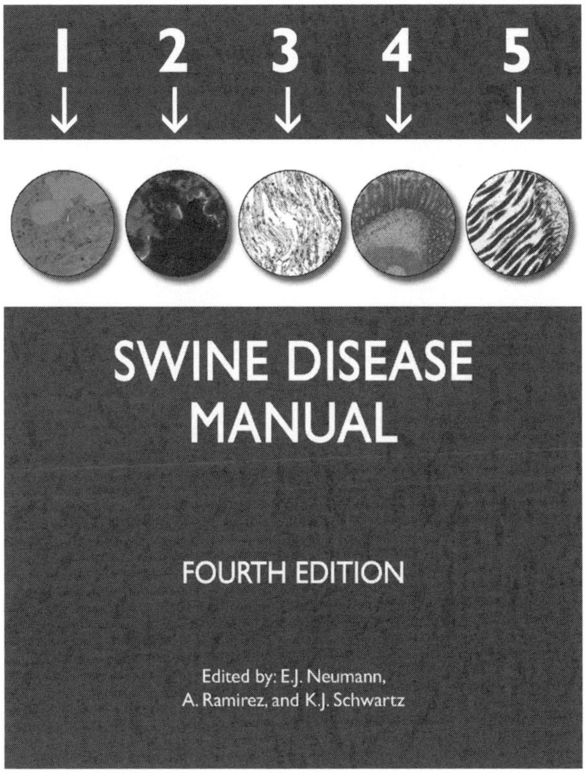

Front Cover

1. Lung: Immunohistochemistry positive for PCV2 antigen

2. Lung: Fluorescent antibody technique positive for *Mycoplasma hyopneumoniae*

3. Heart (aborted piglet): Immunohistochemistry positive for PCV2 antigen

4. Colon: Superficial necrosis and exudation of neutrophils after infection with *Clostridium difficile*

5. Colon: Electron micrograph of the "end on attachment" of *Brachyspira pilosicoli*

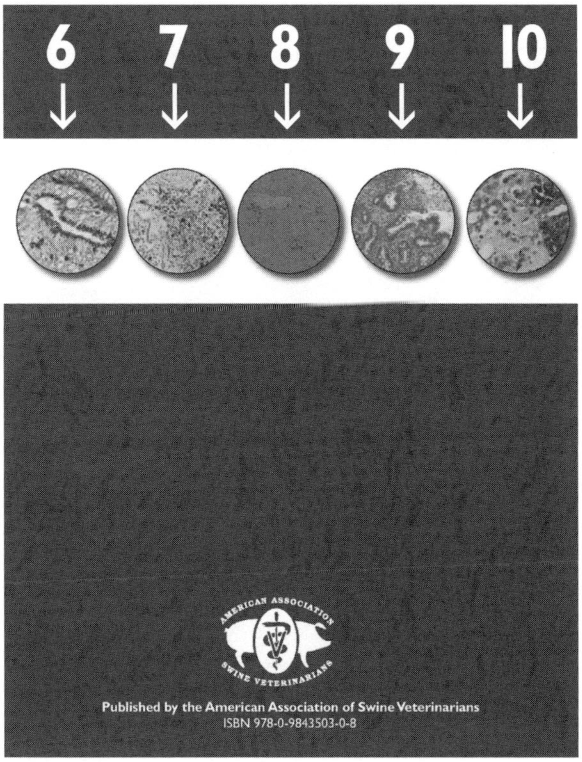

Back Cover

6. Ileum: Silver stain positive for *Lawsonia intracellularis* organisms

7. Lung: Immunohistochemistry positive for PRRSV antigen in macrophages

8. Liver: Immunohistochemisty positive for PCV2 antigen staining

9. Colon: Ulceration and suppuration following infection with *Clostridium difficile*

10. Intestine: Gram's stain demonstrating necrosis with large Gram-positive rods (*Clostridium perfringens* type C)

Photos courtesy of Iowa State University Veterinary Diagnostic Laboratory staff.

PREFACE

This manual was written primarily for veterinary students and those who teach swine diseases. It also may be of interest to veterinary practitioners, veterinary technicians, and others interested in swine diseases in production systems. This manual attempts to update, condense and simplify the great mass of information available. Only basic material appropriate for students is included. More detailed information is available via an array of texts, websites, and scientific publications.

Disease topics are listed as individual entities. The student should be reminded that in reality, the occurrence and severity of disease outbreaks are strongly influenced by production practices, housing, environment, nutrition, and genetics. Diseases may occur concurrently in modern production systems with large populations of animals; for example, porcine respiratory disease complex (PRDC) is usually a co-infection with *Mycoplasma hyopneumoniae* and/or other bacteria or viruses. Diagnostic methods for disease complexes are usually more complicated than finding a single agent. Likewise, control of disease frequently involves not only specific intervention, but also modification of environment, husbandry, and production practices. For this reason, the prevention and control sections in this manual refer to specific agents but are not always appropriate or complete in terms of control of disease complexes. Swine practitioners expend considerable effort in diagnosis, herd investigation, and understanding the interactions of risk factors before implementing cost-effective control strategies. These activities are beyond the scope of this manual but our vision is that this manual will serve as a foundation on which to build a better understanding of the complexities of disease in swine populations.

Familiarity with the organization of the manual will make it more useful. The table of contents lists the diseases and conditions of swine covered in this manual. Most sections are based on the nature of the etiologic agent, and all are preceded by their own table of contents. The time-saving index at the back of the book lists each major disease by name, often cross-referenced with a synonymous name.

A section on exotic (foreign to the US) diseases is provided for ready reference. Any of these diseases may be introduced to the US as a consequence of international trade in swine, pork products, and other contacts. A basic knowledge of these diseases is a good defense against US epidemics.

Several tables are included. Some are designed to help in differential diagnosis. Others list major diseases of a single body system and permit a rapid overview of diseases of that system. The tables may be of special value in preparing for board exams.

Comments on the manual and how it can be made more useful are encouraged and appreciated. They can be mailed to Dr. Kent Schwartz, 1642 Veterinary Medicine, Iowa State University, Ames, Iowa 50011 or e-mailed to **kschwart@iastate.edu**.

Table of Contents

Section I

Diseases Caused by Bacteria, Mycoplasmas and Spirochetes

Actinobacillus pleuropneumoniae (APP)

Definition
This organism causes severe pleuropneumonia which is a highly contagious disease of swine often characterized by sudden onset, short clinical course, high morbidity, and high mortality.

Occurrence
Porcine pleuropneumonia (PPN; currently referred to as APP) is widely distributed throughout major swine-raising countries. It has been a major problem in many European countries and is relatively common in the United States, Canada and Asia. APP is restricted to swine. In naïve herds, APP occurs in all age groups but usually is seen in 6-20 week old pigs. *Actinobacillus suis* can cause similar disease and lesions but is not as contagious as *Actinobacillus pleuropneumoniae* (APP).

Historical information
In the United States, APP was first reported in 1957. It was reported frequently in the 1960s and 1970s. Frequency of outbreaks increased with the industrialization of swine production. Research has been greatly facilitated by use of infected seeder pigs to reproduce APP under experimental conditions. Because of the economic consequences of disease, most producers strive to eliminate infection from herds.

Etiology
The etiologic agent of APP is *Actinobacillus* (previously *Haemophilus*) *pleuropneumoniae*. The organism is a hemolytic, Gram-negative, capsulated, coccobacillary rod, highly host-specific for swine. Strains vary in virulence and pathogenicity. There are two biotypes distinguished by their dependency for NAD (nicotinamide adenine dinucleotide) in culture. Within the two biotypes, at least 15 serotypes are commonly recognized; four (1, 3, 5, 7) are most common in North America. The organism does not persist for any significant time in the environment.

The APP organism secretes 4 exotoxins, ApxI, ApxII, ApxIII and ApxIV, together called RTX toxins, and produces abundant endotoxin. The RTX toxins are cytotoxic and/or hemolytic. The toxins produced vary among the 15 serotypes. Antibodies to the exotoxins probably are important in protective immunity.

Actinobacillus suis is closely related to *A. pleuropneumoniae* and some strains produce one or more of the RTX toxins. The two organisms may cross react on some serologic tests.

Epidemiology
Swine that survive acute APP often remain carriers. Swine can also be subclinically infected carriers with only occasional disease outbreaks. Most transmission is by direct contact of APP via nasal secretions but transmission may be via aerosol, at least for short distances. Overstocking, inadequate ventilation, coinfection with other respiratory pathogens, or unusual stress may facilitate transmission or precipitate outbreaks. Fomites, including boots and coveralls, can spread the organism but are infectious for only a short time.

Pathogenesis
Hemolysin and other toxins produced by APP are active against endothelial cells and pulmonary alveolar macrophages. Presumably, they also cause a vasculitis in the lungs and at other sites. Vasculitis precedes thrombosis and is followed by infarction and sequestration of infarcts in the lungs. Sudden deaths may be caused by endotoxic shock.

Pathogenesis probably involves both variable host resistance and various degrees of virulence among serotypes. Generally, serotypes 1 and 5 are considered more virulent than 7 or 3 but all can cause significant disease and any of these may be present subclinically in populations of pigs.

Other pathogens or environmental factors that affect the lung may influence onset and course of the disease. Colostral immunity in young pigs confers some resistance to infection and permits gradual development of active immunity in many exposed, growing pigs. Naïve pigs suddenly exposed to APP are more likely to develop fulminating clinical signs.

Clinical signs
Signs vary considerably between acute and chronic forms of APP. In acute outbreaks, sudden deaths are common. The early signs include sudden onset of prostration, high temperatures, apathy, anorexia, stiffness, and perhaps vomiting and diarrhea. A shallow, nonproductive cough is occasionally present. As disease progresses, there is marked dyspnea with mouth breathing and, perhaps, a foamy, bloody discharge from the mouth and nose. There is early peripheral cyanosis of extremities. As circulation fails, generalized cyanosis follows. Morbidity and mortality in growing swine varies but can become high. Peak mortality usually occurs in pigs 10-16 weeks old. Mortality can reach 20-80% in fattening pigs. Abortions may occur in acutely infected pregnant females.

Chronic cases may become apparent following an acute outbreak. Chronic cough and slow growth then are the usual signs due to the presence of pleural adhesions and abscesses that form in recovered lungs.

Lesions
Lesions of APP are usually restricted to the respiratory tract; characteristic lesions include necro-hemorrhagic areas of consolidation in the lung accompanied by fibrinous pleuritis. The thoracic cavity often contains blood-tinged fluid. The classic lesion is hemorrhage and necrosis in the dorsal portion of one or both diaphragmatic lobes. Lesions in the lungs are dark red to black, firm, and develop as areas of infarction. Bloody froth often fills larger airways and there may be interlobular edema. Fibrinous pleuritis almost always overlays pneumonic areas and extends to adjacent costal pleura.

There may be serofibrinous pericarditis. Pharyngitis, sometimes necrotic and ulcerative, may be present. Occasionally there is polyarthritis.

Chronic cases often have large, sequestered or encapsulated nodules of necrosis in the lungs that incompletely resolve as abscesses. Lung lesions often are attached to the rib cage by fibrous adhesions which lead to condemnations at slaughter.

Accurate differentiation of APP and *Actinobacillus suis* on the basis of lesions is difficult, perhaps impossible.

A. suis infection more often is accompanied by bacteremia with involvement of other organs making bacterial culture an important tool in establishing a diagnosis. Disease caused by *A. suis* tends to be more sporadic and less severe but this organism can cause substantial disease in naïve or "high health" populations. Also in finishers and older animals, cutaneous lesions that resemble those of acute erysipelas are reported with *A. suis*.

Diagnosis

The sudden onset of an acute, rapidly-spreading, respiratory disease causing high morbidity and mortality is suggestive of APP. Dark red infarcts in the lungs of acutely affected cases, sequestered nodules in lungs of chronic cases and a high incidence of pleuritis in the herd also are suggestive. Virulent serotypes exist within both biotype I (NAD dependent) and biotype II (NAD independent). Isolation and identification of APP is confirmatory. A culture technique using immunomagnetic separation has been described for isolating the organism from mixed bacterial populations. Polymerase chain reaction (PCR) techniques targeting the RTX toxin genes are also available and can facilitate differentiation from *A. suis* infection.

Despite limitations of specificity, the complement fixation (CF), enzyme-linked immunosorbent assay (ELISA), or hemolysin neutralization serology tests also are useful for diagnosis of APP on a herd basis. They help in identifying infected herds and serotypes in a locality. Low antibody titers to APP in only a few pigs may have little diagnostic significance.

Acute outbreaks of APP must be differentiated from other respiratory diseases, especially *A. suis* infection, pneumonic pasteurellosis, pneumonic salmonellosis, influenza and mycoplasmal pneumonia.

Control

Herds on premises free of APP should be managed as closed herds since introduced swine may be carriers. Swine necessarily introduced should be from APP-free herds. They should be introduced only after testing before and following a quarantine period of at least 30 days.

Management factors of importance in prevention include all in/all out production with careful cleaning and disinfection between farrowings, avoidance of overstocking, proper ventilation, and elimination or control of predisposing diseases.

A new generation of vaccines, cross protective for all serotypes, has been developed. They are subunit vaccines based on the use of purified and, in some instances, outer membrane proteins. They should not interfere with the serologic tests that use capsular or lipopolysaccharides (LPS) or polysaccharides.

The older type vaccines are serotype specific. They often are used to increase immunity in the sow herd but routine practice of sow herd vaccination remains controversial. Vaccination of piglets should be delayed until piglets are 5-7 weeks old and maternally derived antibodies are depleted. Some autogenous bacterins contain stabilized hemolysin and may be of benefit.

A novel vaccination approach based on intranasal inoculation of baby piglets has recently been developed in Australia. Results of early work with the product look promising but only limited experimental work has been presented to support its distribution to a world-wide market.

Usually, control of APP in endemically infected herds requires combinations of vaccination, medications and improved husbandry. In some cases, the best efforts fail to control disease effectively. Often, the cost of long-term control is unacceptably high.

If APP is endemic in a sow farm, depopulation can be a cost-effective approach to eradication of the disease. Depopulation should be followed by thorough cleaning and disinfection of the buildings and leaving them vacant for a few weeks; restocking can then follow using APP-free swine. As possible alternatives, APP may be controlled in the offspring by early weaning or medicated early weaning at no more than 17 days of age. Important caveats include first boosting immunity in the sows using serotype-specific antigens, assuring that piglets received adequate amounts of their colostrum, weaning to a clean site, and good biosecurity.

Acute outbreaks demand immediate parenteral antimicrobial treatment of affected animals and those in adjacent pens. This, combined with the addition of antibiotics in feed or water for a few weeks, can reduce mortality. Commonly used agents used for prevention and/or treatment include tiamulin, tulathromycin, chlortetracycline, ceftiofur, tilmicosin, florfenicol, enrofloxacin and procaine penicillin G. Many strains are resistant to tetracyclines. Chronic cases usually are unresponsive to treatment.

Actinobacillus suis

Definition

An infectious disease characterized by hemorrhages and embolic lesions at multiple sites, more obviously in the lungs, and often by serous or serofibrinous exudates in the thorax and abdomen.

Occurrence

Outbreaks occur predominantly in immunologically naïve populations. These include primary and secondary specific pathogen free (SPF) pigs or in segregated early weaned (SEW) pigs. Most outbreaks are in recently weaned pigs and in grow/finish pigs derived from an SEW system. Outbreaks occur in both younger and older swine and, less often, in conventionally raised pigs.

Historical information

There have been reports of the disease since 1962. In the 1980s, after management techniques were introduced that minimized exposure of neonates to many endemic pathogens, the incidence of *Actinobacillus suis* infections appeared to increase in the US industry. Misdiagnosis of the disease as *Actinobacillus pleuropneumoniae* (APP) infection or other septicemias likely contributes to underreporting of the true prevalence of the disease.

Etiology

The etiologic agent, *Actinobacillus suis*, is only now being studied in detail. It is a Gram-negative, nicotinamide adenine dinucleotide (NAD)-dependent, non-motile coccobacillus. It is aerobic and facultatively anaerobic. All isolates appear to be of a single serotype. Strains from swine appear to be clearly different from those isolated from horses.

Thus far there is no serologic test to reliably identify infected swine and establish *A. suis*-free herds. Antibodies to *A. suis* and *A. pleuropneumoniae* may cross-react with some serologic tests.

Epidemiology

The epidemiology is not completely understood but carrier pigs probably introduce *A. suis* into herds. It can be isolated from the nasal cavity and tonsils of many healthy pigs and has been found in the reproductive tract of healthy sows. It is believed to be an "early colonizer" of neonates. Less than optimal environmental conditions or concurrent diseases may increase the ability of *A. suis* to cause disease.

Pathogenesis

Invasion probably occurs through the tonsil and spreads through the bloodstream. This is suggested by the presence of the organism in emboli in the vasculature at many lesion sites. The agent's pathogenic effect is probably a result of production of hemolysin and other toxins similar to those produced by *A. pleuropneumoniae*.

Clinical signs

The first signs of an outbreak may include sudden death of young pigs with lesions attributed to a bacterial septicemia. Sick piglets are febrile, breathe rapidly, and may have congested or cyanotic extremities. Cyanosis, arthritis, enteritis, and rarely necrosis of the feet, tail and ears have been reported and are similar to other causes (streptococcal, erysipelas, salmonella) of bacterial septicemia. Occasionally, infected pigs may show central nervous system (CNS) signs including tremors, shaking or paddling. Mortality within affected litters can be high, up to 50%.

Older growing pigs and adults can have similar signs but may also have signs of acute respiratory distress. Lethargy or depression, anorexia, and rarely irregular reddened skin lesions that resemble those of erysipelas may be observed. Pregnant sows may abort.

Lesions

Lesions are similar in pigs of all age groups. They include petechial and ecchymotic hemorrhages in many organs. Frequently, lesions are present in the lungs as disseminated foci of hemorrhagic to necrotizing pneumonia, the latter more marked in older piglets and growers. A consistent lesion in all age groups is serous or serofibrinous exudate in the abdominal and thoracic cavities. Polyarthritis may occur in grow/finish pigs.

Microscopic lesions occur in many major organs. These develop around small colonies of *A. suis* within the vascular emboli or thrombi. Occasionally there are eosinophilic clubs surrounding the colony. Both gross and microscopic lesions are typical of embolic, bacterial septicemias.

Diagnosis

History, signs and lesions are suggestive of the diagnosis but it should be confirmed by culture of *A. suis* from multiple organs. Serologic diagnosis is unreliable because antibodies to *A. suis* and APP may cross react.

Control

Autogenous vaccines have been used but have not been evaluated critically. Because there are multiple types of lipopolysaccharides (LPS) in *A. suis*, the LPS profile of the vaccine strain must match that of the pathogen. Although unproven, vaccines against APP may offer some cross-protection.

Actinobacillus suis is sensitive to many antibiotics including ampicillin, amoxicillin, oxytetracycline and others. Sick pigs should be treated parenterally as soon as possible. The exposed group can be treated by medicating the water.

Anthrax

Definition
Bacillus anthracis can cause an acute bacterial disease in most warm-blooded animals, including swine and man.

Occurrence
In swine, anthrax is relatively rare except when large numbers of anthrax organisms are ingested. Although anthrax occurs throughout the world, incidence in swine in the United States is low. Anthrax in grazing animals other than swine tends to occur in certain geographic areas and to be seasonal. This may not be true of swine.

Historical information
Although there are many old reports on anthrax in species other than swine, most reports on the disease in swine have occurred since 1952-53. At that time a major epidemic occurred in several Mid-western states. The outbreak was caused by imported, contaminated bone meal used in preparing feed for swine. The feed was widely distributed before anthrax was finally diagnosed.

In 1989-90 an outbreak lasting over 14 weeks in a 500-sow operation was reported. Reports on this outbreak serve to emphasize the great difficulties and expense in depopulating, cleaning and disinfecting a large contaminated confinement facility or slaughterhouse.

Etiology
Anthrax is caused by *Bacillus anthracis*, a large, aerobic, Gram-positive rod. The organism is easy to culture and nonhemolytic colonies appear on blood agar in 12-18 hours. Colonies have irregular borders and are sticky when touched by a bacteriologic loop. Under suitable aerobic conditions, spores are formed and are quite resistant to heat, desiccation and many disinfectants. Spores can persist in favorable soils for over 15 years.

In tissue the organisms have a well-developed capsule and grow in short chains. They have square ends where in contact with others of the same chain but may be rounded on free ends.

Epidemiology
Decaying, anthrax-infected carcasses and their fluids contaminate the soil where resistant spores are then formed. Most grazing animals ingest the spores while grazing over contaminated soil. Swine, however, are rather resistant to anthrax and seldom are infected while grazing. Infection of swine usually occurs when they have fed on an anthrax-infected carcass or when feeds containing large numbers of spores are fed to them. The source in contaminated feeds is the animal source component, e.g. bone meal, tankage or meat scraps.

Pathogenesis
During infection the anthrax bacilli produce a complex exotoxin. A lethal factor in the exotoxin is responsible for the death of experimental animals and, presumably, of swine. Lethal factor causes depression of the central nervous system (CNS) and has a harmful effect on mitochondria.

Invasion of the anthrax bacilli usually is through defects in the pharyngeal mucosa or the tonsils. Invasion often is followed by lymphangitis and localization of *B. anthracis* in tonsils and/or cervical lymph nodes. Alternatively, there can be focal or multifocal localization in the intestine followed by spread to one or more mesenteric lymph nodes. Localizations tend to be necrotizing. Frequently both pharyngeal and intestinal lesions develop. There seldom is a septicemic form of anthrax in swine except, perhaps, in young pigs.

Clinical signs
Sudden, unexpected deaths may be the first signs of anthrax following a highly variable incubation phase (one to 20 days). Signs depend upon the site of localization of lesions. Three forms of anthrax, based on site of localization, are termed pharyngeal anthrax, intestinal anthrax, and septicemic anthrax. Swine with pharyngeal anthrax, the most common form, show marked cervical swelling and dyspnea; they may die from suffocation. Other signs include fever, depression, and inappetence, perhaps vomiting.

Swine with intestinal anthrax have similar signs except that cervical edema and dyspnea may not be apparent. Also, there may be bloody feces. Both pharyngeal and intestinal forms can occur in the same animal. Swine are fairly resistant to anthrax and spontaneous recovery from cases with localized lesions is not unusual. Septicemic cases have a short course and may result in sudden death.

Lesions
A necropsy should not be performed on any animal suspected of having died from anthrax; spores will be formed when the carcass is opened and will persist at the site. Necropsy also will expose humans to anthrax.

In anthrax-infected cadavers, rigor mortis may be weak or absent and the blood may fail to clot. Many animals have no visible external lesions other than, perhaps, pharyngeal swelling. Animals with pharyngeal anthrax, opened inadvertently, usually have a gelatinous cervical edema and markedly enlarged, hemorrhagic, cervical lymph nodes. Tonsils often are covered with fibrinous exudate. There may be a marked pharyngitis. In chronic cases, necrotic lesions in nodes or tonsils may be grayish yellow and circumscribed; often these (signs) are seen in recovering animals.

Swine with intestinal anthrax usually have peritonitis with excessive, bloody peritoneal fluid. Fibrin may be present in the fluid and overlay the serosa of affected segments of intestine. The mesentery attached to affected intestine is edematous and may contain reddened streaks around the vasculature. There are focal or multifocal areas of severe, often diphtheritic, enteritis. Regional lymph nodes draining the area are enlarged and reddened. Animals with intestinal anthrax often have pharyngeal lesions.

In septicemic anthrax, more likely in small pigs, carcasses appear pale and dehydrated. There is bloodstained peritoneal fluid and scattered petechiation.

Diagnosis

Although bacteremia and septicemia are unusual in swine with anthrax, it is advisable to take a peripheral blood sample aseptically for smears and culture. Smears can be fixed in Zenker's solution and stained with polychrome methylene blue. Anthrax bacilli will appear as long, square-ended, blue rods with a pinkish capsule. Alternatively, smears can be stained with Gram stain. The large Gram-positive, rod-shaped organisms have a "boxcar" appearance that is presumptive but not definitive, of anthrax. Sometimes it may be necessary to biopsy or excise an affected lymph node for culture, using sterile technique. Any necessary cut on a suspected cadaver should be disinfected or plugged with a mass of cotton saturated with 10% formaldehyde.

B. anthracis can be cultured on blood agar and identified from colonies that soon develop. If in doubt about identity of the colony, or if the culture is not pure, it may be possible to purify the culture and confirm the diagnosis by scarifying and inoculating the footpad of a laboratory mouse or guinea pig. They will develop anthrax and the bacillus can then be isolated in pure culture from the laboratory animal. Anthrax must be differentiated from pharyngeal malignant edema, acute erysipelas and CSF.

All cultures, contaminated materials, disposable equipment and infected experimental animals and their feces should be incinerated. Any known or suspected areas of contamination should be disinfected. Ten percent fresh sodium hydroxide, 5% formaldehyde, and 2% glutaraldehyde are among the better disinfectants for *B. anthracis*.

Control

An attenuated live vaccine against anthrax has been used for prevention in some species but is seldom used for swine since they have enough natural resistance to withstand considerable exposure. Limited experience seems to indicate the vaccine could be used to advantage if necessary. Prevention in swine is usually by avoidance of heavy exposure that might occur through ingestion of anthrax-infected carcasses or contaminated feeds. Laws now exist that prevent importation of raw bone meal. Some states have laws that regulate the use of animal origin products in feeds.

Treatment of infected animals can be effective if given early. Both penicillin and oxytetracycline have been used effectively.

Atrophic Rhinitis (Progressive Atrophic Rhinitis)

Definition

An infectious disease characterized in early stages by snuffling, sneezing, snorting, and perhaps nosebleed which may progress to atrophy and distortion of the turbinates, nasal and facial bones of some affected pigs.

Occurrence

Atrophic rhinitis (AR) is restricted only to swine although a similar disease has been described in dogs and goats. Signs and/or lesions can occur in any age group of swine more than one week old. In the United States, AR is becoming a rare disease as prevalence has been decreasing in most areas as a result of early weaning, age segregation and/or vaccination. AR occurs in all major swine-raising countries.

Historical information

Atrophic rhinitis (AR) was described first in 1830. AR was reported in the US in 1944. It rapidly increased in frequency with expansion and intensification of swine production and stimulated a great amount of research. AR has a complex etiology.

Etiology

Toxigenic strains of *Bordetella bronchiseptica* and *Pasteurella multocida* (primarily type D) may cause AR. *Bordetella bronchiseptica* is an aerobic, Gram-negative rod. The organism readily colonizes the nasal passages of swine and is widely distributed in the swine population. It often is non-pathogenic but can sometimes cause severe losses from septicemia and suppurative bronchopneumonia in pigs up to 12 weeks old. *Bordetella bronchiseptica* has been isolated from many species other than swine (dogs, cats, rodents, rabbits, wildlife). Those strains are not believed to play a role in causing AR in swine. However, toxigenic porcine strains can cause atrophy of turbinates, particularly in pigs one to six weeks old. Lesions tend to be mild and can be largely repaired by the host, therefore may not lead to progressive AR.

Toxigenic *Pasteurella multocida* is less widespread in the swine population. Colonization of the nasal passages is enhanced following prior insult to nasal mucous membranes. It often can be isolated from tonsils and lungs of swine with or without the usual signs and lesions of AR. It sometimes is found together with *B. bronchiseptica* in outbreaks of AR. Toxigenic *P. multocida* produces a potent dermonecrotizing toxin that causes marked turbinate atrophy as well as bony alterations in nasal and facial bones. Turbinate lesions usually are initiated in pigs less than 16 weeks old but older pigs can be affected if immunologically naïve. The lesions can persist for a lifetime.

Management and husbandry factors have long been suspected of being important predisposing or contributing factors to AR. Research on dust in confinement houses suggests the incidence of AR may be increased by three toxic agents; endotoxin from Gram-negative bacteria; beta 1, 3-glycan, a cell wall component of molds; and possibly peptidoglycans from cell wall components of all bacteria. More research is needed in this area.

Epidemiology

Numerous factors assure survival of toxigenic *B. bronchiseptica* and *P. multocida* among swine. Atrophic rhinitis results in the establishment of inapparent carriers. Swine introduced into a clean herd from an outside source can be carriers and disseminate the agents that cause AR. Also, carrier sows expose their piglets. When their infected piglets are mingled with others, the agents can be transmitted. Although immune sows provide their piglets with some colostral immunity against the agents that cause AR, waning colostral immunity and weaning soon leave young pigs susceptible to infection. Older sows may provide more colostral immunity (and perhaps less infective dose) than do gilts. Several microbiologic agents, other than *B. bronchiseptica* and *P. multocida* are known to cause or be associated with rhinitis (see Diagnosis). The rhinitis they cause may predispose to colonization by the bacteria that cause AR. Management or environmental factors, when slighted or ignored, increase the susceptibility of pigs to AR. Ventilation is an especially important factor. Irritating dust or ammonia from urine and feces may contribute to the severity of rhinitis. The irritants make nasal mucous membranes more susceptible to colonization by the primary agents of AR. Other contributing factors include overstocking, substandard housing or sanitation, continuous use of facilities, and failure to use all in/all out production methods.

Pathogenesis

There is colonization of the nasal passages by toxigenic strains of *Bordetella bronchiseptica* and/or *Pasteurella multocida*, perhaps augmented by environmental or other microbial irritation of turbinates. *Bordetella bronchiseptica* adhere to the nasal mucosa, probably by attaching to the ciliated epithelial cells. The toxin elaborated by the organisms diffuses into the turbinates and is responsible for an osteopathy and hypoplastic rhinitis. Later, after the disease becomes more quiescent, some degree of regeneration and repair can occur. The term "regressive atrophic rhinitis" sometimes is used for this form of AR.

Toxigenic *P. multocida* colonizes the nasal mucosa, probably after a rhinitis has been established by *B. bronchiseptica*, other agents or environmental irritants. Toxigenic P. *multocida* produce a potent toxin that causes a rhinitis with progressive osteopathy of facial and turbinate bones. The term "progressive atrophic rhinitis" sometimes is used to indicate this form of AR.

Clinical signs

Signs may appear in pigs as young as one week old but more often appear shortly after weaning. Sneezing, snorting and a serous or mucopurulent nasal discharge are early signs of AR. Rhinitis obstructs the flow of tears through the infraorbital ducts and tears flow from the medial canthus of the eyes causing "dirty" or discolored hair and skin below the canthus. Signs caused by *B. bronchiseptica* alone tend to peak in a few weeks, and then diminish. Signs related to toxigenic *P. multocida* often appear in four to eight week old pigs and may persist for weeks or months. Signs occasionally include nosebleed in more acute outbreaks in weaned, growing pigs. Growth retardation may become apparent. Occasional pigs develop secondary bronchitis, bronchiolitis or pneumonia as an indirect effect of AR.

A variable number of pigs develop lateral or dorsal deviation of the snout. Dorsal deviation often results in shortening of the snout or wrinkling of the skin over the snout. Marked snout deviation in many pigs usually is associated with toxigenic *P. multocida*.

Lesions

Lesions are usually restricted to turbinates, nasal septum and nasal and facial bones and can be observed by sawing transversely across the snout at the commissure of the lips (2nd premolar or 1st cheek tooth in pigs less than 6 months of age). Lesions vary in severity and are usually graded on a scale of 0-5. Minor lesions must be differentiated from normal variations in anatomy and breed character.

Mild lesions usually result in atrophy of the ventral scroll of the ventral turbinates; severe cases are more likely to involve the dorsal turbinate scrolls. In extreme cases the dorsal and ventral turbinates may be almost completely destroyed and there may be atrophy of ethmoid turbinates. Deviation of the nasal septum is more common in severe cases. Nasal and facial bones may be thinned or distorted. Mucoid or mucopurulent exudate often is present on blanched mucous membranes and in adjacent sinuses. Microscopic study usually reveals fibrous replacement of the bony plates of conchae that remain.

Diagnosis

History, signs and lesions often are adequate for a clinical diagnosis of AR, with confirmation by isolation and identification of the etiologic agent(s). Bacterial cultures made from nasal swabs from live or sacrificed pigs are most rewarding early in the course of infection (nursery).

Differential diagnosis should exclude other diseases or irritants that can cause rhinitis such as porcine reproductive and respiratory syndrome virus (PRRS), pseudorabies virus (PRV), inclusion body rhinitis (cytomegalovirus), or excessive dust or ammonia.

Control

After the specific cause(s) of AR have been accurately determined and the extent of loss considered, a decision should be made to either attempt to control the disease, or to depopulate and restock with swine known to be free of AR. If the decision is made to control rather than eradicate AR, control measures fall into three major categories. The first control measure is improvement of husbandry, management and housing, including ventilation. The second measure is initiation of a vaccination program for the breeding stock, pigs, or both. Vaccination of the sows may be most cost effective. Sows often are vaccinated twice at about four and two weeks prior to parturition. Bacterin-toxoid vaccines provide some protection and historically were widely used. The third control measure involves administration of antibiotics to sows and piglets around the time of farrowing/weaning in an effort to limit the extent of colonization in the young pigs. The value of antibiotic therapy to control AR in growing swine is questionable.

Progress of controlling AR should be evaluated repeatedly by examining the nasal passages of a substantial number of swine submitted for slaughter. Several systems for scoring the severity of lesions are available.

Eradication of toxigenic *P. multocida* from a herd or system has been successful. The method first combined medication and pre-farrowing vaccination of sows. Later, their litters were medicated and early weaned at 8-10 or 12-14 days. Finally, nasal swabs were used on maturing animals, toxigenic *P. multocida* isolates were identified by polymerase chain reaction (PCR) testing, and infected animals were identified and eliminated.

Brucellosis (Swine Brucellosis)

Definition
An infectious disease of swine characterized by reproductive impairment or failure and often by localization of *Brucella suis* in bones and joints of breeding stock.

Occurrence
Swine brucellosis (SB) occurs primarily in domesticated swine with feral swine and possible wild hares as potential reservoirs of infection in some countries. The disease occurs in many countries where domestic or feral swine are present in large numbers.

Swine brucellosis once was common in the United States but now, due to rigorous control measures, is unusual in the US. The porcine type of brucellosis occurs as a serious zoonosis, primarily among abattoir workers, farmers and veterinarians.

Historical information
Brucellosis was first identified as a disease of swine in 1914 but was believed to be a form of bovine brucellosis caused by *Brucella abortus*. In 1919 the porcine organism was named as a separate species (*B. suis*). Swine brucellosis increased in importance as swine production intensified and because of the severe disease caused in people. A cooperative, 3-stage, State-Federal-Industry eradication program was initiated with a goal of eradication of brucellosis. This goal is nearly accomplished in domestic herds, but feral swine remain a reservoir in the US.

Etiology
Under the present classification scheme *Brucella suis* is the organism that causes most brucellosis in swine. There are 5 biotypes of *B. suis*. Biotypes 1 and 3 cause generalized infections that result in reproductive failure.

Brucella suis organisms are moderately resistant to environmental influences. Survival time of organisms in the environment decreases as temperatures rise. However, the bacteria often survive desiccation and can survive freezing and near-freezing temperatures for over two years. Pasteurization of milk kills *B. suis*. Most commonly used disinfectants, as well as ultraviolet light, kill the organism.

Epidemiology
Brucella suis usually is transmitted to susceptible swine through direct contact with infected swine. The route of exposure ordinarily is through the alimentary or genital tract. Pigs often are infected by ingesting aborted fetuses, fetal membranes or fluids discharged at the time of abortion. The organisms are also transmitted in infectious semen during natural breeding and artificial insemination. Transmission through abraded skin, conjunctiva and nasal mucous membranes is possible.

Cattle can be infected naturally with *B. suis*. Milk and aborted fetuses can transmit the organisms to swine. Milk-borne epidemics have occurred in people and swine. Infected feral swine, if in contact with domestic swine, are another source of exposure.

The bacteremia that occurs during infection of swine often results in infectious carcasses. Abattoir workers can be infected through handling infectious carcasses or cuts of meat. Farmers and veterinarians may be exposed while assisting sows at farrowing or while handling infectious placentas or newborn, infected piglets.

The prolonged survival of *B. suis* in hog lots and farrowing houses probably is a significant factor in the spread of infection, especially in colder climates or seasons on those premises where management and sanitation are poor. Swine moved into infectious lots or buildings can be infected by surviving *B. suis*.

Pathogenesis
Penetration of mucous membranes by *B. suis* results in colonization of regional lymph nodes, either in lymph or within macrophages. Colonization in regional lymph nodes is followed by long, continuous or intermittent periods of bacteremia. The bacteria then infect and persist in many other organs, including lymph nodes, placenta, mammary gland, joint fluids, bone and in the testicles or accessory genital organs of boars.

A large percentage of swine, especially the females, recover after several months. The recovery rate in boars is low, perhaps never more than 50%. Enough animals remain infected in a herd to perpetuate the disease. Surprisingly, most piglets in infected herds are free of infection at the time of weaning.

Clinical signs
Most owners of *B. suis*-infected herds notice no signs of infection prior to evidence of infertility in the herd. In dams infected at breeding, disease is first suspected when numerous sows or gilts return to heat 30-45 days after breeding. Females first exposed during late gestation have abortions or dead and weak pigs. Early abortions often go undetected.

Sows and gilts usually recover promptly after aborting, successfully re-breed, then deliver live pigs. Infected boars present few signs of infection although their fertility may be below normal. They may or may not show lack of sexual drive.

Lesions
In dams, gross lesions are limited except in chronic cases. At the time of abortion, there may be some degree of endometritis. (Miliary endometritis occurs in *B. suis* type 4 infection in Europe). Occasionally, some of the fetal membranes are retained. Infected placentas may not have grossly visible lesions or may be congested, edematous and have small hemorrhages. Infected fetuses may have subcutaneous edema, especially around the umbilicus, and there may be effusions in body cavities.

Chronic infections in breeding stock may be manifested as fibrinous or fibrinopurulent arthritis. These lesions often affect the large joints of the legs. Osteomyelitis may be apparent within vertebrae, especially the lumbar vertebrae, sometimes with paralumbar abscesses present.

Microscopic lesions include small granulomas in the liver during the bacteremic phase of acute infection. Small, focal areas of inflammation, or microabscesses, may be found at many sites, including the bone marrow adjacent to the epiphyses of long bones. The microscopic lesions are suggestive of brucellosis but not specific.

Diagnosis

Diagnosis usually is made on the basis of serologic testing. The buffered, acidified plate antigen (BAPA) test and the standard card test (SCT) have been used extensively as presumptive tests. For confirmation, either the standard tube test (STT) or the particle concentration fluorescence immunoassay (PCFIA) is used. Serologic testing is very useful as a herd test but is not infallible on individual animals.

All testing for swine brucellosis has limitations. Swine may be infected for 6-8 weeks before developing antibodies that will result in a positive test. In uninfected herds, occasional animals that test positive will later test negative. Infections with several other genera of bacteria may result in positive brucellosis tests. In particular, infection of swine with *Yersinia enterocolitica* has led to positive tests for brucellosis. The limitations of testing sometimes are justification for a slaughter program as part of an eradication effort.

Direct culture probably is the most accurate and sensitive method of diagnosis of acute cases but usually is less practical than serologic testing. Specimens include lymph nodes from slaughter, blood, semen, castrated testicles, infected joints, vaginal swabs or aborted materials from suspect cases. The bacteriologist should be alerted if brucellosis is suspected since colonies are slow-growing and easily missed in routine diagnostic investigations.

Control

Prevention is best accomplished by focusing on implementation of those measures that are most likely to prevent exposure. No animals should be added to a herd without having originated from a negative herd. Those animals should test negative initially, be quarantined for at least a month, then again be tested and negative before being added to the herd. No effective vaccines are available for immunization of swine.

Infected herds can be handled in two different ways. If the herd has many reactors, as is often the case, the premise should be depopulated and allowed to stand idle for at least 2-3 months before restocking. This often is the least expensive way. Depopulation with slaughter of infected herds is often used in the final efforts at eradication. If a herd test reveals only one or a few reactors, those can be removed and the herd retested periodically. This approach often fails.

In some cases where valuable bloodlines must be saved, weaned pigs, usually negative when tested at weaning, can be moved to separate, clean premises. They must be retested at least once prior to breeding to tested, clean boars.

Clostridial Diarrhea

Definition

Disease associated with *Clostridium perfringens* (Cp) and other clostridia occur in many different animal species. In swine, three rather common diseases occur. Enterotoxemia associated with *C. perfringens* type C (CptC) is characterized by variable morbidity and high mortality in neonates or suckling pigs with sudden deaths, bloody diarrhea, or necrotic enteritis. Neonatal diarrhea is also associated with Cp type A (CptA) but with moderate morbidity and lower mortality compared to CptC. *Clostridium difficile* (Cd) infection of the cecum and colon produces diarrhea with variable morbidity and mortality.

Occurrence

Although most outbreaks of CptC are acute and occur in piglets less than one week old, chronic cases may occur in pigs up to several weeks old. The disease has been reported in many other countries. Incidence in the United States varies greatly and has been high in certain areas. Type C clostridial enteritis also occurs in young lambs, calves, foals and poultry, less often in adult sheep, cattle and goats.

Diarrhea caused by infection with CptA or Cd has emerged in most developed pig production industries around the world and has coincided with the advent of large, intensive swine production systems.

Historical information

The disease in piglets associated with CptC was reported, reproduced, and researched in the 1960s. Many early reports on CptC enteritis are from species other than swine. Research efforts languished until recent application of gene technologies has allowed further characterization of toxins produced by Clostridium spp. Molecular techniques have also facilitated study and diagnosis of CptA and Cd with particular emphasis on identifying the presence of genes associated with toxin production.

Etiology

Clostridium perfringens is a large, anaerobic, Gram positive bacillus with both vegetative and sporulated forms. Five toxigenic types (A, B, C, D, E) are distinguished by major toxins they produce (alpha, beta, epsilon, or iota); all types produce alpha toxins. Use of polymerase chain reaction (PCR) technique to detect the genes coding specific toxins has simplified their identification. Type C organisms produce several toxins, especially a necrotizing beta toxin which causes the severe necrotizing enteritis. *Clostridium perfringens* type A produces alpha toxin and those pathogenic for swine also produce beta2 toxin. CptC causes much milder enteric insult than CptC.

Virulent strains of Cd are known to produce an enterotoxin (TcdA) and a cytotoxin (TcdB) that are associated with both systemic illness in pigs and localized typhlocolitis and mesocolonic edema. See the table, Clostridial Diseases, on page 149.

Epidemiology

Feces from carrier sows contain pathogenic clostridial organisms and, coupled with contaminated farrowing environment, are the likely source of exposure for piglets. The bacteria and its spores survive in soil and can be carried on shoes, boots or other fomites. Each outbreak renews the supply of clostridia in the farrowing environment available to infect the next litter of susceptible piglets. Although other species of animals have CptC infection, there are few reports of interspecies transmission.

Dose and immunity play a large role in disease occurrence. Immune dams (from exposure and perhaps vaccination) likely provide colostral antitoxin immunity to offspring. Sanitation in farrowing rooms between groups decreases the infectious dose in the environment.

Pathogenesis

Clostridium perfringens type C organisms are ingested by piglets within a short time of their birth. Conditions that favor proliferation include absence of acid in the stomach and presence of antitrypsin factor. The clostridia proliferate in the small intestine, attach to epithelial cells and produce necrotizing beta toxin that causes necrosis and desquamation of epithelial cells, accompanied by hemorrhage and severe inflammation. Gas is produced and may accumulate in the lumen and/ or wall (intestinal emphysema). Death ensues as a consequence of mucosal necrosis and the systemic effect of toxins on other organs. In older piglets, clostridial colonization may be secondary to other agents of enteritis, most notably coccidiosis, thus contributing to necrotic enteritis. A similar course of events is likely with CptA, with less tissue insult as the expected outcome.

The pathogenesis of Cd has yet to be entirely described. It likely shares features with CptA and CptC but with effects confined to only the cecum and colon. The role of TcdA and TcdB are important as non toxigenic strains of the organism are commonly found in colonic contents in the absence of any clinical signs or lesions. *Clostridium difficile* enteritis is a common sequelae to long-term oral antibiotic therapy in humans but the disease in swine does not appear to follow this same pattern.

Clinical signs

Clinical signs produced by *C. perfringens* vary depending on infectious dose, virulence, and quantity of antitoxin colostral immunity. Susceptible neonates can become ill in just a few hours after exposure to virulent CptC and may be found dead in as little as 4-8 hours. Sick piglets soon become weak, prostrate and then moribund. Weakened piglets are at high risk of being overlaid by the dam. Piglets with a little more resistance live a few days and may have a bloody diarrhea. Occasionally, piglets may live several weeks, develop a yellow or gray, mucoid diarrhea and remain unthrifty. In acute outbreaks, death can occur even prior to the piglet developing diarrhea. Morbidity is variable but mortality is high, up to 100%, in very susceptible litters.

In uncomplicated CptA infections of both neonatal and weaned pigs, diarrhea is creamy, pasty, or yellow and foamy. Morbidity is high but mortality is generally low. Diarrhea produced by Cd may be indistinguishable from that of CptA or neonatal colibacillosis.

Lesions

In type C infection there may be blackening of the abdominal skin. The peritoneal and pleural cavities may contain excessive, blood-tinged fluid. Typical acute cases have a dark red, necro-hemorrhagic small intestine. The lesions usually involve the entire small intestine but in some cases may be segmental, usually in the jejunum or ileum. The cecum and colon sometimes are affected. Gas, along with bloody fluid, may be present in the intestinal lumen and wall. Piglets that live a few days may have a necrotic pseudomembrane lining the affected intestine. There may be fibrinous serosal adhesions between loops of affected intestine. Microscopy reveals necrosis with severe suppurative inflammation; organisms in close association with epithelium will also be evident.

Gross lesions are unremarkable with CptA and consist of thin-walled, fluid-filled small intestine. Microscopically, there are often accumulations of neutrophils at villus tips, perhaps with necrosis or sloughing of apical enterocytes. Occasionally, sporulating rods are detected in close association with enterocytes.

Clostridium difficile lesions are confined to the cecum and colon, and include moderate to severe mesocolonic edema, watery colonic contents, and occasionally respiratory symptoms or sudden death. Microscopic erosion of the colonic epithelium with infiltration of mononuclear inflammatory cells is a common finding.

Diagnosis

The acute, short course with high morbidity and mortality and typical gross lesions in neonatal piglets are highly suggestive of type CptC enteritis. Identification of a large population of Gram-positive, rod-shaped bacteria in mucosal smears is strongly supportive of the diagnosis. Identification of exceptionally large numbers of *C. perfringens* in anaerobic cultures from small intestine is helpful. Although seldom necessary, a number of laboratory techniques are available to identify the necrotizing beta toxin in intestinal content from typical cases. Diagnosis can be markedly strengthened by microscopic study of intestinal lesions which are nearly pathognomonic for type C infection. Specimens should be selected from acutely affected pigs early in the course of disease.

Type A infections usually have much milder gross and microscopic lesions, nonbloody diarrhea and lower mortality. Clostridial enteritis must be differentiated from other neonatal diarrheal diseases, including colibacillosis, rotaviral enteritis, transmissible gastroenteritis (TGE) and particularly, coccidiosis.

The PCR technique is now being used in some labs to separate clostridial genotypes C and A. Presence of identified toxic genes correlates closely with production of toxins. An isolate from a typical case may be used to determine the type of infection.

Diagnosis of Cd can be a difficult task but always involves a combination of histopathology, identification of toxin, and culture of the organism.

Control

Immediate passive immunity can be provided for CptC by immune antiserum (antitoxin) given orally or parenterally within two hours of birth. Also, antibiotics effective against clostridia can be given for a few days and may provide some protection.

Considerable protection for piglets (for both CptC and CptA) can be provided by injecting the dams twice with bacterin-toxoid, the first 5-6 weeks and the second 2-3 weeks prior to farrowing. A booster given a few weeks prior to subsequent farrowings is recommended. Where control is less than satisfactory, an autogenous bacterin prepared from an isolate from a typical piglet may be used to vaccinate the sows.

Some benefit may be obtained by feeding antibiotics with anticlostridial activity to sows before farrowing and during lactation. Antimicrobial agents used include bacitracin, tylosin, virginiamycin, lincomycin and others. Commercial bacterin-toxoids are available for both CptC and CptA.

Programs for consistent control of Cd have not been adequately described. Use of strategic antibiotic therapy in piglets and vaccination of dams with autogenous bacterin-toxoid preparations prior to parturition are being explored.

Colibacillosis (*E. coli* Diarrhea)

Definition
Diarrhea associated with *Escherichia coli* can occur in young piglets within a few days of birth through well after weaning. Occasional cases of septicemia are attributable to *E. coli*. Edema disease, a unique form of colibacillosis, is presented separately (see Edema disease).

Occurrence
Colibacillosis affects pigs in all major swine-raising countries. There are many different types of *E. coli*, each of which may possess several of many virulence factors. Many outbreaks occur within the first week after birth. Others occur later during the nursing period. Still others occur about 1-2 weeks after weaning or following abrupt changes in environment or nutrition.

Historical information
Colibacillosis has been recognized as an important diarrheal disease of pigs for over fifty years. For many years treatment and control were largely empirical. Recurring losses, as well as the importance of *E. coli* in other species including man, stimulated research on the disease. Research has largely paralleled development of confinement rearing. Advances in molecular biology have simplified specific identification of pathogenic coliforms and their genes related to virulence.

The coliform responsible for several recently reported food poisonings of people, O157:H7, does not appear to cause disease in swine nor is this serotype common in swine.

Etiology
Pathogenic strains of *E. coli* are easily isolated, Gram-negative, flagellated bacilli. Most pathogenic strains form smooth to mucoid colonies; some are beta-hemolytic. Virulence factors include fimbria (pili), enterotoxins (exotoxins), endotoxins, and capsules. Fimbria are the small hair-like processes on the bacterial surface that allow attachment to specific receptors on the surface of mucosal enterocytes of the small intestine (colonization). Pathogenic strains also produce one or more enterotoxins, which are exotoxins elaborated locally in the small intestine that can have either local or systemic effects. These strains are termed enterotoxigenic *E. coli* (ETEC).

There are five common, antigenically distinct pilus types found in pigs: F4 (K88), F5 (K99), F41, F6 (987P) and F18. The first four pilus types mediate adhesion in neonates. F18 is not associated with neonatal colibacillosis but is common in postweaning colibacillosis as is F4. Some strains have the ability to erode epithelium and are termed attaching and effacing *E. coli* (AEEC).

The toxins elaborated by pathogenic *E. coli* in swine (ETEC) are labile toxin (LT), stable toxin A (StA), stable toxin B (StB), and verotoxin (shiga-like toxin, SLT). The first three act locally causing hypersecretion of fluid from the intestine while verotoxin is responsible for the systemic vascular effects of edema disease (discussed separately).

In summary, there are many strains and types of *E. coli* present in swine and their environment. Enteropathogenic *E. coli* require the presence of both fimbria-mediated adhesion to enterocytes as well as elaboration of one or more toxins.

Epidemiology
Potentially pathogenic *E. coli* are present in the intestinal tract and feces of many normal swine. Dams often act as immune carriers. Continuous farrowing, accompanied by poor sanitation and chilling, can increase the risk of colibacillosis. *E. coli* organisms contaminate the skin and mammary glands of dams and are ingested by nursing piglets. Piglets with little colostral or inherent immunity (enterocyte receptors for certain pilus types are not present in all genetic lines of swine) sicken first. Pathogenic coliforms are magnified by fecal shedding to further increase exposure of littermates. Disease occurrence and severity is related to dose ingested and the level of immunity derived from colostral immunity.

Pathogenic coliforms survive in contaminated buildings and can infect successive litters of pigs. Once present, *E. coli* tend to persist unless vigorous efforts are given to maintaining sanitation, husbandry, and environment.

Pathogenesis
Ingested pathogenic *E. coli* adhere to receptors on microvilli of enterocytes via pili. There they colonize, proliferate, and elaborate enterotoxins that cause excessive secretion of fluid and electrolytes by crypt epithelial cells which markedly exceeds absorptive capacity resulting in a net flow of tissue fluids into the lumen. Up to 40% of a piglet's weight may be lost as fluid passed into the intestine. The enterotoxins, endotoxin, and/or adhesins may damage the microvilli and enterocytes as well. This reduces the absorption of electrolytes, water and endogenous secretions from the lumen. The large intestine, sometimes also affected, is unable to absorb the excess fluid and diarrhea results. Damage to epithelial cells sometimes leads to septicemia. Diarrhea usually continues until death results from dehydration and metabolic acidosis or from terminal septicemia.

Post-weaning colibacillosis is similar but with one additional consideration. Verotoxigenic strains elaborate verotoxin (shiga-like toxin) which has systemic effects on endothelium of blood vessels (edema disease). These strains are sometimes hemolytic on blood agar.

Whether piglets contract colibacillosis depends on a balance between the number and virulence of pathogenic *E. coli* in the intestine, the pigs' resistance to the disease, and environmental factors (temperature, humidity, sanitation, etc.). Neonatal piglets have incompletely developed immune systems and limited innate resistance. They are largely dependent on antibodies supplied in colostrum and milk. Anything that prevents piglets from obtaining colostrum leaves them susceptible to colibacillosis.

If purchased gilts farrow before they have developed antibodies to endemically present pathogenic *E. coli*, their colostrum and milk may not contain enough antibodies to protect their piglets. Also, as the nursing period progresses, piglets get less milk and the milk contains fewer antibodies. Chilling of piglets impairs intestinal motility and lowers resistance to infection. Massive exposure can overwhelm resistance. In recently weaned pigs, absence of milk antibodies and the different type of feed may contribute to outbreaks of colibacillosis.

Clinical signs

Colibacillosis usually is signaled by the appearance of diarrhea. Piglets from gilts may be more severely affected than piglets nursing sows. The severity of the diarrhea varies. The hypersecretory diarrhea usually has an alkaline pH but varies in color. It may be clear and watery, especially in neonates, but may be white or yellow, influenced by type of ingesta and duration of the disease. Sick pigs occasionally vomit but vomiting is not as prominent as with transmissible gastroenteritis (TGE).

As diarrhea continues, there is progressive dehydration and the hair coat becomes roughened. Body temperature often is subnormal. Shivering often is noted unless an adequate supplementary heat source, such as heat lamps, is available. Signs are similar in pigs of various ages but tend to be more severe in younger pigs. Death losses can be severe if husbandry and environmental conditions are poor. Diarrhea tends to persist until intervention is accomplished.

E. coli is one of the most common causes of neonatal septicemia and polyserositis. Often, strains associated with septicemia are not enteropathogenic.

Lesions

Dehydration is the most obvious clinical sign. The small intestine and colon may contain excess watery fluid or may be distended and gas-filled. There may be mild reddening and congestion of the stomach. Lesions often are surprisingly mild, especially in very young piglets. However, in outbreaks caused by certain pathogenic strains, usually in older postweaned pigs, there can be marked congestion of the gastrointestinal tract.

Microscopy of the mucosa of the small intestine reveals many coliforms adhered to microvilli of intestinal epithelial cells. Villi usually are intact. With some strains of *E. coli*, there may be necrosis of some villi and microvascular thrombosis in the lamina propria.

E. coli is a common cause of septicemia in neonates. In those cases, there is fibrinous polyserositis and arthritis.

Diagnosis

Typical signs and lesions are useful but not definitive. The isolation of a uniform and high population of smooth, mucoid, or hemolytic *E. coli* from the small intestine is suggestive of colibacillosis. Diagnostic labs often use one of the following methods to more specifically identify the pathogenic *E. coli*:

- A slide agglutination test can identify the serogroup but does not confirm pathogenicity.
- Adhesin(s) can be identified using monoclonal antibodies.
- A polymerase chain reaction (PCR) can identify the pathogen genetically. Genotyping by multiplex PCR is widely practiced to determine specific pilus and toxin genes present in the isolate.

Diagnostic methods do not identify important contributing factors such as chilling, poor sanitation or starvation. These often must be corrected if prevention or treatment is to be successful.

Colibacillosis has to be differentiated from other diarrheal diseases of young pigs. These include transmissible gastroenteritis (TGE), rotaviral infection, coccidiosis and *Strongyloides* parasitism. Starvation is also a major differential diagnosis.

As *E. coli* are commonly found in the small intestine of both normal and diseased pigs, microscopic examination of small intestinal sections can be useful in distinguishing the significance of the infection. Dense colonization of the brush border with adherent *E. coli* should be expected in most cases of colibacillosis with additional erosive or congestive changes present depending on the toxins that have been elaborated.

Control

Many experienced veterinarians believe that colibacillosis is related largely to problems in housing and management which cause the disease secondarily. More detailed information on housing and management is available elsewhere. A few general guidelines on prevention and treatment follow:

Insofar as is possible, breeding stock should be obtained from a single source with no problems of colibacillosis. Dams should be acclimatized together for 3-6 weeks prior to breeding and during gestation so they can develop immunity to endemically occurring pathogens. This allows for the production of an adequate amount of specific antibodies in colostrum and milk.

It often is worthwhile to try to enhance the immunity of sows by using vaccines made from bacterial pili or toxins or both. Pregnant dams often are vaccinated twice at 2-3 week intervals prior to farrowing. A recent analysis of the value of vaccination, based on data from a National Animal Health Monitoring System (NAHMS) national survey, predicts that *E. coli* vaccination of sows would be cost effective for producers.

Another method of increasing colostral antibodies is feeding some farrowing house waste to sows during late gestation. Waste should include any pathogens present in the farrowing house and will stimulate formation of antibodies against them. Oral vaccination of sows with virulent *E. coli* cultured in milk was quite useful prior to the development of commercial injectable vaccines.

Use of the all in/all out system of raising piglets is recommended. Farrowing should occur in a facility thoroughly cleaned, disinfected, and dried between farrowings. The build-up of pathogens can be minimized by a vigorous, ongoing sanitation program.

The farrowing facility should be designed to provide a dry, comfortable environment for both dams and piglets. This requires lower temperatures (~70° F) for sows and areas warmed (to ~90° F) for small piglets. Stresses on piglets should be minimized.

When precautionary efforts fail, a system should be available to treat piglets immediately if signs of colibacillosis appear. Antimicrobials can be administered to neonates orally or by injection. Due to the contagious nature of the organism, when treating sick pigs before weaning, all pigs (including those not scouring) in the litter also need to be treated at the same time. Weanlings can be given antibiotics in water. Antimicrobial sensitivity data is quite useful in selection of an appropriate antimicrobial. Oral electrolyte replacement solutions sometimes are used to help control dehydration. Various products may aid in prevention of postweaning colibacillosis. Plasma proteins, zinc oxide, organic acids, and probiotics are commonly used.

Some swine are genetically resistant to certain fimbriae of pathogenic *E. coli*. Breeding for genetically related resistance eventually may help control some forms of colibacillosis.

Edema Disease (read chapter on Colibacillosis first)

Definition

An acute, often-fatal enterotoxemia of recently weaned pigs caused by a few serotypes of *Escherichia coli*. It often is characterized by edema at certain sites, sudden deaths, and occasionally by neurologic signs related to lesions in the brain.

Occurrence

Edema disease (ED) occurs primarily in recently weaned pigs. It occurs rather frequently in countries that practice intensive swine production. In the US, edema disease is considered sporadic in occurrence, has not been eliminated by modern technologies, and in fact can cause considerable loss in modern production systems.

Historical information

Edema disease is a unique form of colibacillosis first reported in 1938. It was reported only occasionally during each of the next two decades. Following World War II, swine production was intensified and highly nutritious rations were introduced. The frequency of ED then increased. Much of the present information on ED is the result of research completed during the last 25 years.

Etiology

Edema disease is caused by toxins produced in the small intestine by pathogenic serogroups of *Escherichia coli* (*E. coli*). Most have pilus type F18 or F4 (K88), and elaborate shiga-like toxin (variably referred to as SLT-IIe, Stx2e, verotoxin, edema disease principal, neurotoxin, or vasotoxin). Enterocyte receptors for pili are genetically determined and variably present, depending on genotype of the pig. Purified Stx2e given intravenously to experimental pigs results in typical edema disease. Other forms of colibacillosis (diarrhea) can be caused by some of the same pilus types that cause ED but have a different pathogenesis because of the variety of enterotoxins that may be elaborated.

Epidemiology

Because outbreaks of ED in nurseries sometimes occur repeatedly, pathogenic serogroups probably persist in the environment of the farrowing rooms and/or nursery or are reintroduced by carrier dams.

Several factors appear to influence the bacteria that cause ED. Specific enterocyte receptors are a function of pig genotype. Some receptors are not present until postweaning. Maternal antibody in colostrum and milk may be a factor. Nutrition also plays a role since ED occurrence can be influenced by ration type and frequency of feeding. High protein diets, certain dietary constituents, and rotavirus may make the intestine more favorable for colonization of enteropathogenic *E. coli*.

Pathogenesis

Pathogenic *E. coli* colonize and proliferate in the small intestine by pilus-mediated attachment to the epithelial cells. Enterotoxins produced by pathogen strains induce the disease, with Stx2e causing damage to small arteries and arterioles. Degenerative angiopathy leads to increased vascular permeability and accumulation of edema at various sites, most notably colon, stomach, small intestine, eyelids, and brain. Damage to vessels in brain can cause malacia in the brain stem and basal ganglia, a feature in subacute stages of the disease having central nervous system (CNS) disturbance. High doses of Stx2e may cause acute hemorrhagic gastroenteritis or sudden death.

Clinical signs

Onset of the disease usually is around two weeks postweaning. Onset often is signaled by finding a few thrifty pigs dead. Morbidity usually is low but mortality is high in pigs that show signs. Signs include anorexia, ataxia, stupor and recumbency often accompanied by paddling and running movements. When caught, affected pigs may respond with an abnormal squeal, a consequence of laryngeal edema. Diarrhea usually is not present in pigs with typical ED but may be present in other pigs in the same group. Swelling of the face and eyelids may or may not be present. Sick pigs die within a few hours or days. The few that survive often have neurologic deficits. The course of ED in a herd usually is around two weeks. However, the disease may reappear as other batches of pigs reach the age group at risk.

Lesions

Several affected pigs should be necropsied since not all will show typical lesions. In some pigs found dead, congestion of viscera may be the only appreciable gross change. Usually, some will have evidence of edema of subcutis of the face or eyelids, gastric submucosa, or in the mesentery of the spiral colon. Fluid may be increased in the peritoneal cavity, chest or pericardial sac. Occasionally there are hemorrhages under the epicardium or endocardium. The brain may have unique hemorrhagic and malacia lesions in brain stem or basal ganglia in less acutely affected pigs. These lesions are very suggestive of ED.

In subacutely or chronically affected pigs, microscopic degenerative changes can be found in small arteries and arterioles at many sites. The changes sometimes are apparent in vessels supplying the brain. Histologic sections of brain stem and basal ganglia may confirm suspected areas of hemorrhage and malacia.

Diagnosis

The history, signs and lesions often are adequate for a tentative diagnosis. Bacterial culture of the small intestine from a nonmedicated typical pig will yield high populations of hemolytic colonies of *E. coli*. It is useful to genotype the isolate for confirmation of virulence factors and perhaps for epidemiologic reference. Typical microscopic vascular lesions help confirm diagnosis.

Edema disease must be differentiated from other causes of neurologic signs (pseudorabies, water deprivation or organic arsenical poisoning) or septicemia and meningoencephalitis caused by *Streptococcus suis*, *Salmonella* serotype Choleraesuis, erysipelas, or *Haemophilus parasuis*.

Control

Treatment of pigs affected with ED can be frustrating since toxin production in the gut is quite advanced by the time clinical signs become visible. Affected pigs must be treated parenterally. Antimicrobials may be of some value in less severely-affected pigs. Supportive therapy to counteract acidosis and dehydration is valuable in early cases. During an outbreak, efforts are directed toward reducing the incidence of infection in the remainder of the population at risk. Administration of antimicrobials and acidifiers in the water may be helpful. In severe outbreaks, removing feed and replacement with a ration containing less protein, a lower percentage of soybean meal, or higher proportion of rolled oats is required.

No prevention method is universally accepted or successful because the erratic occurrence of ED makes intervention strategies hard to assess. Seven general strategies should be considered when formatting control strategies for affected farms.

1. Management factors include minimizing environmental stresses (e.g. temperature variation, drafts, damp conditions), limited commingling, and using all in/all out (AIAO) system with scrupulous sanitation.
2. Nutritional considerations include creep feeding, restricted feeding, multiple feedings (small quantities 3-6 times/day) after weaning, adding oats (high in fiber) to the rations, acidifiers (organic or inorganic acids) added to feed or water, decreased protein in the ration, addition of zinc oxide (2500 ppm) to the ration, and addition of plasma protein.
3. Antimicrobial intervention is often practiced. Various antibiotics have been added to rations or water but the efficacy is difficult to evaluate because outbreaks do not occur regularly; some affect only a few pigs, some pigs are naturally immune, and outbreaks end spontaneously. Antimicrobial resistance eventually dooms this strategy over the long term.
4. Immunoprophylaxis can be successful by passive or active protection. Oral ingestion products (milk, plasma protein, egg powder) containing antibody can help to prevent colonization and disease. Disadvantages of passive protection are cost, lack of cross-protection between pilus or toxin types, and possibility of susceptibility remaining following cessation of feeding. Active immunity can be induced against specific adhesins or toxins. Oral vaccination with live or killed cultures that contain F18 or F4 (K88) pili but lacking genes for toxin production have been successful. Toxoids prepared from Stx2e have also been demonstrated effective against ED but are not commercially available. Whole-cell bacterins have been much less effective.
5. Competitive exclusion, a process whereby receptors for *E. coli* are occupied by nonvirulent agents, is being investigated and may offer opportunity for control in the future.
6. In herds negative for ED, it is prudent to prevent introduction by careful scrutiny of disease history of breeding stock. Eradication may be possible by using depopulation and disinfection.
7. Natural resistance to ED is possible in pigs genetically lacking receptors for F18 and/or F4 (K88) pili. Genetically resistant pigs have been developed.

Erysipelas (Swine Erysipelas)

Definition

Erysipelas is an infectious disease mostly of growing or adult swine. It may be clinically inapparent, may cause acute illness involving many animals, or be a chronic disease characterized by enlarged joints, lameness, and endocarditis. Rhomboid skin (diamond-skin) lesions are an inconsistent feature only associated with acute cases.

Occurrence

Erysipelas occurs in swine, lambs and turkeys. It occurs occasionally in other poultry and many kinds of wild birds. Seasonal distribution has not been documented but losses may be greater during warm summer months. Sporadic outbreaks are seen in most kinds of livestock, wild mammals (including rodents), reptiles and amphibians. Erysipeloid, a localized skin infection, occasionally occurs in people who work with infected animals or process meats, poultry, fish or animal by-products. In humans, the disease referred to as "erysipelas" is actually caused by a streptococcal infection.

Historical information

In 1885, Dr. Theobald Smith isolated an organism from swine in the US that was similar to one Pasteur had isolated 3 years earlier from swine with *rouget du porc*; both were eventually identified as *Erysipelothrix rhusiopathiae*, the causative agent of swine erysipelas (SE). In 1886 Dr. Friedrich Löffler, a German bacteriologist, published the first accurate description of SE.

In the US, SE did not assume importance until 1928 when several outbreaks were reported in South Dakota. Within a few years, erysipelas began to be reported frequently from many geographic regions. Prevalence of SE decreased after introduction of bacterins but remains a constant threat, unaffected by widespread adoption of confinement rearing.

Etiology

Erysipelothrix rhusiopathiae is a Gram-positive, aerobic, slightly bent, thin bacillus. It is resistant to many environmental influences and survives for long periods of time in pork meats, cured hams, contaminated fish meal and decaying animal carcasses. There are at least 26 serotypes of which swine are susceptible to at least 15. In the United States, most isolates from sick pigs are serotype 1a, followed by 2, 5, and 1b. Nonpathogenic species (*E. tonsillarum*) have been isolated from normal swine. The organism is sensitive to penicillin and usually to tetracyclines. It resists many antibiotics and sulfonamides. It can be destroyed by many disinfectants, including caustic soda and hypochlorites.

Epidemiology

Erysipelothrix rhusiopathiae is thought to be spread among swine by carriers in the herd. Many healthy swine are carriers of pathogenic and/or nonpathogenic *Erysipelothrix* and disseminate the organism in their feces and oronasal secretions. Pigs affected with erysipelas also shed large numbers that contaminate feed, water, soil and bedding. Contaminated soil probably does not remain infective for more than 35 days. The resistant organisms can flow in surface water to adjacent premises. A wide range of wild mammals, poultry, wild birds and pets can disseminate the bacteria. There is empirical evidence that biting flies and ticks can sometimes transmit *E. rhusiopathiae* between swine. The many carriers of *E. rhusiopathiae* make eradication of SE unlikely.

Pathogenesis

Ingestion of contaminated feed and water usually allows *E. rhusiopathiae* to gain access to the body, probably through the tonsils or other lymphoid tissue of the digestive tract (the organism often can be cultured from tonsils of normal swine). Less often, contaminated skin wounds may permit entry. In acute erysipelas, and perhaps in other forms of the disease, a bacteremia develops and leads to spread of organisms throughout the body.

The precise mechanism by which *E. rhusiopathiae* causes disease is speculative. The organism produces neuraminidase, an enzyme that cleaves mucopolysaccharides in cell walls which may mediate the widespread vascular damage that accompanies SE. Vascular damage leads to thrombosis and interference with microcirculation in capillaries and venules at many sites.

In chronic arthritic cases, there is a vasculitis with exudation of fibrin into perivascular tissues and joint(s). There also is marked villous proliferation of the synovial membrane. Joint lesions are more proliferative than exudative. Pannus may develop and eventually result in destruction of articular cartilage and ankylosis of adjacent bones. Connective tissue formation around joints is stimulated, apparently by perivascular fibrin, and the joint capsule may be thickened. Persistence of inflammation around an affected joint may be from a few living bacteria in the joint or it may be the result of hypersensitivity to remaining bacterial antigens.

Vegetative, valvular endocarditis, another manifestation of chronic erysipelas, is less common than joint involvement. Emboli of *E. rhusiopathiae* are believed to cause inflammation of blood vessels within heart valves. In the inflammatory process, the endocardium is breached and bacterial colonies are established at the site. Fibrin is deposited there and slowly organized to form nodular vegetations. Emboli that arise from vegetations can cause sudden death. Interestingly, outbreaks of vegetative endocarditis can occur in the absence of other clinical signs.

Susceptibility to infection is not well understood. Many swine known to have been exposed to organisms do not sicken with the disease. Lactogenic immunity protects piglets for several weeks. In older, susceptible swine, various stresses (heat, aflatoxin, poor nutrition) have been suspected of playing a role in precipitating outbreaks.

Clinical signs

Swine erysipelas will be discussed as acute or chronic erysipelas. However, clinically inapparent erysipelas probably occurs and may precede acute or chronic SE.

Many acute outbreaks of SE occur in animals approaching market weight. Acute outbreaks often begin with the sudden and unexpected death of one or a few thrifty pigs. Careful observation then reveals other sick pigs with very high temperatures (104-108°F), usually without respiratory signs or diarrhea. Sick pigs often have reddened or cyanotic skin, especially about the ears, snout, jowls, throat and ventral abdomen. On a few of the animals there may be discrete, raised, and red to purple areas of skin. These often have a rhomboid or diamond shape and are more obvious on white pigs. On dark skinned pigs, the lesions may be visible or palpable as slightly raised patches of hair. Leg joints are painful but may or may not be swollen. Affected pigs resist getting on their feet but are alert. When forced to arise, they often have to be assisted, squeal with pain, stand with their feet close together and soon lie down again. Pregnant sows may abort.

Classic cutaneous rhomboid urticaria (diamond skin) occurs in a percentage of pigs shortly after the acute febrile stages. Cutaneous lesions may coalesce over the rump, back or shoulders. Large patches of skin may have sloughed or still be attached to underlying, healing areas. Sloughing of the tip of the tail or tips of the ears can occur with chronic erysipelas but can have other causes. In younger pigs (suckling, nursery, grower) with acute erysipelas, signs are similar, with cyanosis of extremities, ears and snouts pronounced and urticaria less common.

The chronic forms of SE may follow acute outbreaks or develop insidiously. SE frequently is manifested by enlargement of joints in an increasing number of pigs, often with little mortality. Chronic SE, when manifested by cutaneous lesions, more often follows acute outbreaks. Pigs with valvular lesions in the heart often present few signs unless exerted. They then may show respiratory distress, perhaps collapse and die.

Lesions

Pigs which die of acute erysipelas may present as "sudden deaths" and may not have discrete gross lesions. The cyanosis or diamond-shaped skin lesions will remain apparent. Necropsy may reveal congested lymph nodes, often quite edematous; there may be subcapsular hemorrhage if the animal lived a few days after onset. Petechial hemorrhages may be present on the kidneys, epicardium and endocardium. The liver is swollen and the capsule tense. The lungs frequently are congested and edematous. The spleen may be markedly enlarged, especially in cases that lived a few days; it occasionally may contain infarcts.

Chronic, arthritic cases have a proliferative, villous synovitis in one or more swollen joints (hocks or carpal). Synovial fluid is viscous and only modestly increased in amount. The joint capsule may or may not be visibly thickened. An organized inflammatory exudate (pannus) may be present in affected joints, sometimes with ulceration of the articular cartilage or ankylosis of adjacent bony surfaces.

Chronic cutaneous lesions may be apparent as one or more patches of dry, necrotic skin. Sometimes there are granulating, healing areas where patches of necrotic skin have sloughed.

Vegetative, valvular endocarditis of chronic cases usually affects the mitral valve and may appear as irregular masses of considerable size. Such cases often have infarcts in the spleen, kidneys or other sites, the result of embolism from valvular lesions.

Microscopic lesions include vasculitis in capillaries and venules at many lesion sites, including glomerular tufts, pulmonary alveolar walls and skin. *E. rhusiopathiae* bacteria may be apparent within microthrombi in blood vessels.

Diagnosis

Clinical diagnosis is based on signs, typical lesions in several pigs and favorable response of acute cases to high doses of penicillin and/or hyperimmune serum. Pigs in the early stage of acute erysipelas often respond favorably; severe or chronic cases do not. In acute cases, signs of special value in diagnosis include exceptionally high temperatures, evidence of marked pain in multiple joints and typical skin lesions. Diagnosis can be confirmed by bacterial culture of kidney, spleen, lymph nodes, blood, or other tissues and, where available, polymerase chain reaction (PCR). Culture of *E. rhusiopathiae* is more likely from acute cases; failure to recover the organism should not rule-out a diagnosis of erysipelas. Acute erysipelas must be differentiated from acute hog cholera and acute septicemia (salmonellosis, streptococcal infection). *Actinobacillus suis* is also reported to cause cutaneous lesions that resemble those of acute SE.

A firm diagnosis is more difficult with chronic cases. Culture attempts on multiple joints often fail. However, the appearance of many cases of arthritis in growing pigs is more typical of erysipelas than of other diseases. Vegetative, valvular endocarditis can be caused by many different organisms, most notably *Streptococcus suis.*

E. rhusiopathiae should be cultured from those vegetations before diagnosing chronic SE.

Control

Acute outbreaks of SE usually can be controlled by administering penicillin and/or erysipelas antiserum to affected pigs along with antimicrobials added to the drinking water until no sick pigs have been observed for at least three days. Vaccination in the face of an outbreak is warranted.

A vaccination program is advisable for premises on which outbreaks have occurred or where exposure is expected. Attenuated vaccines and bacterins are available with recent products improved, having duration of immunity of 26 weeks and efficacy across a broad spectrum of serotypes. Killed vaccines may be given by injection and attenuated live vaccines via injection or in drinking water. Two doses of most bacterins usually will protect growing pigs to market weight but may have to be boostered later in grow-finish stages in some herds, especially those with a history of repeated exposure to the organism. Booster vaccination at least 1-2 times per year is recommended for breeding stock.

A combination of regular vaccination, good sanitation, the elimination of carriers with skin and joint lesions, and appropriate quarantine measures for purchased stock usually will aid control of SE.

Greasy Pig Disease (Exudative Epidermitis)

Definition

An acute, exudative dermatitis of pigs from a few days to about eight weeks of age characterized by variable to high morbidity and variable mortality.

Occurrence

Exudative epidermitis (EE) occurs in most major swine-raising countries. It is a sporadic disease, one occasionally seen by most swine practitioners. Although acute EE usually occurs in pigs less than eight weeks old, including nursery pigs, the disease also occurs in a less severe form in older pigs. It seldom occurs in adult swine and then is manifested only as a few localized lesions. A similar dermatitis, "greasy heel," occurs on the pasterns of horses. The same agent that causes EE can be isolated from the pastern lesions. However, there is no proven transmission from horses to pigs.

Historical information

Exudative epidermitis was described over 150 years ago. Subsequently, it was reported under a variety of names. *Staphylococcus hyicus*, the etiologic agent, was first identified as a staphylococcus in 1965 and differentiated from nonpathogenic staphylococci in 1978. Despite research, the complete etiology of EE is unclear.

Etiology

Staphylococcus hyicus, a Gram-positive coccus, is the etiologic agent. At least six serotypes have been identified. There are differences among strains isolated from pigs and other animals. In swine, *S. hyicus* has been isolated from many sites, including the skin, nasal mucosa, vagina and prepuce. Under experimental conditions certain strains have reproduced the disease. Typical lesions of EE also have been produced by a bacteria-free supernatant from the agent. Five exfoliative exotoxins that target cells of the stratum granulosum in the epidermis have been identified; both toxigenic and non-toxigenic strains exist. EE may be caused by an exotoxin alone although predisposing factors probably play some role.

Many predisposing factors for EE have been suggested. These include vesicular viral diseases (certain strains of parvovirus, poxvirus, perhaps an unidentified virus), nutritional deficiencies (zinc, vitamins), ringworm infection, pityriasis rosea, parasitism (including lice infestation), housing inadequacies, immunologic inadequacy of young pigs (especially in litters from gilts), lack of competing bacterial flora on the skin, poor hygiene, poor ventilation, high humidity, initial abrasions of the skin from trauma, and genetic susceptibility.

Epidemiology

The epidemiology is unclear. *S. hyicus* is present in many herds and yet causes no disease. Under experimental conditions, only certain strains can colonize the skin and cause disease. Some outbreaks have followed the introduction of swine from other herds. Others have not, so that other risk factors (trauma, environmental irritation) are likely involved. The disease is more frequent in new or start-up herds or when a large number of gilts are being introduced into an established herd. One can only speculate that one or more of the predisposing factors listed above precipitate outbreaks.

Pathogenesis

Initial skin lesions are focal erosions in the stratum granulosum. Lesions extend into hair follicles and lead to a suppurative folliculitis. Sebaceous glands secrete excessively and there is accumulation of greasy exudate over lesions. There soon is severe epidermal erosion and ulceration. Exudate on the surface dries and deep cracks and fissures develop. Lesions enlarge and may coalesce. Degeneration and sloughing of renal epithelium often occurs, possibly the result of dehydration. Deaths are related to dehydration, loss of serum proteins and electrolytes.

Clinical signs

Listlessness or depression and anorexia are early signs and may involve part or all of a litter. Body temperatures seldom are elevated. Although the skin is reddened, there is no pruritis. Initial lesions may occur in the axilla or groin but often go unnoticed. Brownish spots, one to two centimeters in diameter and covered by serum and exudate, appear on the skin of the face or head. The lesions later appear as brown to black crusts. In acute cases the lesions enlarge and coalesce, spread from the head posteriorly and may generalize within 24 to 48 hours. Although initial lesions usually affect haired areas, ulcers may develop on the tongue or in the mouth.

Young pigs can die within 3-5 days. Overall morbidity and mortality usually are high in younger pigs. Pigs older than about eight weeks may have only a few lesions, largely confined to the head. They often survive but tend to gain weight slowly. Adult swine occasionally have a few brown exudative lesions on the back and flanks. Lesions on adults are uncommon and often unrelated to known outbreaks in younger pigs.

Lesions

At necropsy the affected pigs usually are dehydrated and malodorous. The lesions observed clinically may be quite extensive and vary in number and severity among pigs in the same litter. The crusts often are fissured and contain dirt and filth from the environment. In chronic cases there may be inflammation of the external ears. Lesions are predominantly on haired areas, including the feet, but may affect the mouth and tongue. There may be linear streaks on renal papillae, and ureters and kidney pelvises may contain cellular debris. Occasional pigs have pyelonephritis. Lymph nodes draining the skin are swollen.

Microscopically, there is a pustular dermatitis largely in the stratum corneum and a suppurative folliculitis with bacterial colonies often with suppurative lymphadenitis in enlarged lymph nodes.

Diagnosis

Few swine diseases resemble typical EE. Signs and lesions usually are adequate for diagnosis. Confirmation can be made by isolation of *S. hyicus* or by histopathology. In older pigs with only one or a few localized lesions, EE must be differentiated from sarcoptic mange and other microbial skin infections.

Control

In general, treatment has not been very satisfactory. Injectable antimicrobials may be of some benefit. Anecdotal recommendations have included spraying the pigs several times with solutions such as 10% bleach, chlorhexidine, Virkon® (Durvet) or dilute tamed iodine.

Affected litters or individual pigs should be isolated immediately. Mingling of pigs should be avoided if an outbreak has occurred.

If an outbreak is well established in small pigs before diagnosis, it may be prudent to euthanize those with advanced lesions. Any that recover will gain inefficiently.

Prevention starts with providing a high standard of sanitation for pregnant sows, especially in housing, and washing of sows may be of value. Control of EE may depend largely on preventing trauma and improving the environment with better ventilation, cleaner and drier pens, controlled humidity and reduced stocking density. For prophylaxis, vaccination with an autogenous bacterin of *S. hyicus* has been suggested but results are hard to evaluate since EE is sporadic and may not recur, regardless of vaccination. EE often develops so rapidly that an autogenous bacterin cannot be prepared soon enough.

Haemophilus parasuis (Glasser's Disease)

Definition

An infectious disease of pigs, often acute, characterized by various combinations of meningoencephalitis, polyserositis and polyarthritis as well as a contributor to bacterial pneumonia.

Occurrence

Glasser's disease occurs sporadically among swine herds and is usually observed in three week to four month-old pigs. It often occurs subsequent to stressful events such as weaning, changes in environment, commingling, or as coinfection with other disease agents. Glasser's disease is present in all the major swine-raising countries and remains a significant disease even in modern age-segregated production systems.

Historical information

In 1910, Glasser observed a swine disease and associated it with a small, Gram-negative rod. In 1931 an organism, presumably the same one, was isolated from swine with influenza and named *Haemophilus influenzae suis*. By 1943 it was clear that the organism was a pathogen in its own right, not necessarily associated with swine influenza, and the name was shortened to *Haemophilus suis*. Then by 1976, definitive taxonomic studies resulted in the present name, *Haemophilus parasuis*. The importance of Glasser's disease has increased with expansion of the swine raising industry.

Etiology

Haemophilus parasuis is a small, pleomorphic, and fastidious, Gram-negative rod. It can be grown on blood agar, as satellite colonies, near a streak of staphylococci or source of nicotinamide adenine dinucleotide (NAD). The organism often can be isolated from the nasal cavity or tonsil of normal pigs. It frequently can be isolated from other disease processes, especially pneumonic lungs. As a septicemia, *H. parasuis* has predilection for growth on serosal surfaces (peritoneum, pleura, pericardium, joints, meninges).

At least 21 serovars have been identified with additional untypeable strains also common. Some are more commonly associated with disease than others and groups of pigs often harbor several different serovars. Serovars 4, 5, 13 and 14 are more prevalent in North America. Cross-protection may occur but appears to be incomplete. For example, bacterin prepared from serovars 4 and 5 usually protects against homologous and heterologous 4 & 5 serovars and reduces the number of lesions caused by serovars 13 & 14. Virulence appears to be related to capsular antigens but is not necessarily related to immunogenicity.

Epidemiology

H. parasuis is widely distributed in the swine population and usually causes no disease. Neonatal pigs are exposed to and colonized by the organism early in life. Colostral antibodies usually protect pigs from disease while they gradually develop an active immunity by the time they are 7-8 weeks old. It is presumed that young pigs without either passive or active immunity can develop fulminating disease if exposed to *H. parasuis*. Unusual stresses, such as weaning, prolonged transport or other diseases may predispose to outbreaks.

Pathogenesis

Pathogenesis is poorly understood but vasculitis plays an important role in the development of lesions. *H. parasuis* can be a primary pathogen or be associated with other diseases such as porcine reproductive and respiratory syndrome virus (PRRSV) or swine influenza virus (SIV). Perhaps the lesions or stress of those diseases permit access of the organism. Presumably, there is a period of bacteremia since *H. parasuis* often localizes at multiple sites.

H. parasuis has a predilection for the leptomeninges and brain, often localizes there and stimulates an inflammatory reaction. In addition, the organism often can be isolated from one or more serosal surfaces, often as cause of inflammation and fibrinous exudates. Damage to vasculature, apparent microscopically, probably facilitates formation of inflammatory exudate and increased synovial fluid in joints. The organism is also a contributor to pneumonia by systemic distribution or expanding lesions in typical bronchopneumonia.

Clinical signs

Onset of Glasser's disease is usually sudden. The best pigs frequently are the first affected. They may be found dead or die after a disease course of less than two days. Signs depend upon where the organisms localize. Signs of central nervous system (CNS) disturbance often predominate as a consequence of localization of *H. parasuis* in the brain, meninges and spinal cord. Signs may then include tremors, incoordination, posterior paresis or lateral recumbency. In most cases there is an initial, marked rise in temperature, along with anorexia and depression.

Often there are swollen leg joints (and in some outbreaks arthritis predominates) and the animal will favor an affected leg while walking. Sudden deaths may occur in any age group. There sometimes are signs suggestive of septicemia or myositis. Less frequent signs in all swine include rhinitis, dyspnea, reddening of the conjunctiva, cyanosis of the extremities and edema of the eyelids or ears. Morbidity usually is low but mortality is high among those untreated. *H. parasuis* is also commonly isolated from pneumonic lungs.

Lesions

There may be cyanosis of the skin. Often there is copious serofibrinous or fibrinopurulent exudate in the peritoneal cavity, the pericardial sac or thorax. Pleuritis is a common lesion and may be present with or without obvious pneumonia. Lesions in the lungs often are red, multifocal, disseminated and suggestive of septicemia and hematogenous spread. They closely resemble those of embolic, bacterial pneumonias, especially those caused by *Streptococcus suis*.

Haemophilus parasuis may also contribute to typical bronchopneumonia. The fundus of the stomach often is congested but should be considered a nonspecific lesion. There may be petechial hemorrhages on the kidneys.

Occasionally there are no readily visible gross lesions but if the brain is removed, a fibrinopurulent exudate may be visible on the ventral aspect of the brain. In advanced cases the exudate may be present over the cerebellum or cerebrum. One or more major leg joints often are swollen, perhaps in combination with lesions at other sites. The atlanto-occipital joint frequently is affected. Exudate in joints often is fibrinous and gray to green. An infrequent lesion, recently described, is myositis of the masseter muscles with swelling of the head. Microscopic lesions include vasculitis and fibrinopurulent exudate at lesion sites.

Diagnosis

A tentative diagnosis often can be made on the basis of history, signs and typical lesions. The diagnosis should be confirmed by culture of *H. parasuis* from lesions affecting serous membranes, cerebrospinal fluid, joints or other tissues. Isolates must be differentiated from other *Haemophilus*-like organisms, especially *Actinobacillus suis*. Brain, visceral pleura and other serosal exudates are preferred culture sites. Glasser's disease may involve only a few or many animals in a herd. Consequently, it must be differentiated from numerous other diseases. These include diseases that cause CNS signs, septicemia or arthritis. Molecular techniques for identifying *H. parasuis* from clinical specimens and carrying out epidemiological studies have been well described.

Control

The course of the disease often is short and many of the sick animals die if untreated. For that reason, sick animals should be treated promptly and parenterally with an appropriate antimicrobial. *H. parasuis* is sensitive to many antibiotics and sulfonamides but the sensitivity pattern of isolates from individual farms may vary over time so periodic evaluation of antibiograms is warranted. If numerous pigs are affected, it may be advisable to mass medicate, through the water, all pigs in the affected age group.

Prevention may involve management modifications, sound husbandry, control of primary diseases such as PRRSV, prophylactic antimicrobials, or vaccination. Since *H. parasuis* colonizes relatively early in the piglets' life (less than 10 days of age), segregated rearing has not been uniformly successful in preventing infection or disease. Acclimatization and vaccination of breeding stock has been of some benefit. Minimizing stressors associated with weaning and the nursery environment should be emphasized.

Formalin-killed bacterins are available and can be effective for prophylaxis. Unfortunately, protection against one serovar of *H. parasuis* may not assure good protection against all serovars. Limited research suggests that piglets from dams that have been vaccinated against *H. parasuis* prior to farrowing, or piglets vaccinated when one to three weeks old, have considerable resistance to disease caused by the same serovar. Colostral immunity in the piglets may sometimes interfere with very early vaccination against *H. parasuis* infection.

Recognition of the natural relationship between the infection of young pigs in the face of maternal immunity with subsequent induction of active immunity during this phase has led to innovative approach to control of disease. Preliminary reports suggest that controlled exposure of nursing piglets to live *H. parasuis* organisms indigenous to the farm will allow successful infection and development of active immunity while disease expression is suppressed by maternal immunity. This concept attempts to mimic the natural ecology of organism and host to mitigate disease postweaning.

Leptospirosis

Definition

Leptospirosis is a contagious disease of swine and many other animals (including humans) and is caused by infection with any one of a large group of *Leptospira* spp. serovars. Although the generalities of leptospirosis in swine are presented here, details of infection with different serovars may vary. Swine are susceptible to many different serovars.

Occurrence

Leptospirosis occurs in swine in all parts of the world where conditions are favorable for the survival of leptospires. The occurrence of any one serovar of *Leptospira* in an area depends on the presence of maintenance hosts in which the infection persists or the presence of incidental hosts. In both instances, leptospires can be effectively disseminated to swine. The disease occurs more frequently where the hosts are numerous or concentrated.

Historical information

Early reports of "swine herder's disease" in Europe described a disease among caretakers of swine that probably was leptospirosis. In the US, swine leptospirosis was recognized as an important disease of swine in the 1940s and 1950s. The disease continues to be endemic in areas where environmental conditions are favorable for leptospires. However, losses have been reduced by confinement, sanitation, management changes, vaccination, and the use of antibiotics. Leptospirosis is now relatively uncommon in modern swine production.

Etiology

A new system of classification for *Leptospira* is based largely on DNA relatedness to known reference strains but universal agreement on taxonomy of the genus remains elusive. Under the most current classification, the family Leptospiraceae contains eight pathogenic species of which three are of most importance to swine: *Leptospira interrogans* (serovars *pomona*, *icterohaemorrhagiae*, *canicola*, and *bratislava*), *Leptospira borgpetersenii* (serovars *sejroe* and *tarassovi*) and *Leptospira kirschneri* (serovar *grippotyphosa*). Serovars *pomona* and *bratislava* are uniquely adapted to swine, others are maintained in other species but sometimes infect swine. Of additional note, serovar *L. hardjo* is the most important serovar of bovines and has been reported to infect pigs kept in close contact with cattle. *Leptospira bratislava* is reported to be the most common strain in swine, although the role of this serotype as a cause of disease is debated.

Leptospira are motile spirochetes, 6-12 microns long, and 0.1 micron in diameter. They usually are hooked on both ends and can be stained by Giemsa stain or, in tissue, by silver stains. In the laboratory they often are studied under darkfield microscopy. In laboratory media they are difficult to culture and grow very slowly (12-26 weeks). Many pathogenic strains can survive in the environment for long periods of time under moist conditions with a slightly alkaline pH. Most cannot withstand desiccation and are destroyed by common disinfectants.

Epidemiology

Many of the pathogenic *Leptospira* serovars, including *L. pomona*, have a predilection for the kidneys and persist there. Both maintenance and incidental hosts pass large numbers of *Leptospira* in their urine, often lasting for weeks to months after clinical signs have concluded. Infection usually is introduced into a herd by infected, shedding swine (often replacement gilts or boars), by direct or indirect contact with incidental hosts (rats, mice, skunks, raccoons, foxes, opossums, etc.), or through *Leptospira*-contaminated water, soil, or effluent. Outbreaks have been reported in herds using untreated surface water for drinking.

Under ideal conditions, leptospires survive in water and damp soil. There they remain a persistent threat to a wide range of animals, including swine and man. Incidental hosts can be infected or merely act as passive transport hosts that carry leptospires to other premises. Carnivorous forms of wildlife may visit swine-raising facilities, feed on dead piglets and later visit other premises. They may be underestimated as transmitters of *Leptospira*.

Fetuses infected in utero may survive as infected piglets and, as adult carriers, transmit *Leptospira* to following generations. These inapparent carriers may be selected as replacement breeding stock or sold to other producers. When sold, they can introduce leptospirosis into recipient herds.

Some *Leptospira* serovars, especially *L. bratislava*, have a predilection for the genitalia of both male and female swine. The organisms can be transmitted from infected to negative animals during copulation. In addition, *L. bratislava* can be transmitted through urine.

Pathogenesis

Leptospira penetrate mucous membranes (eyes, mouth, nose, vagina), wounds, abrasions, and perhaps water-softened skin of the host. A leptospiremia then develops and organisms circulate throughout the body and probably affect many major organs. Many species localize in the kidney or in the uterus during the last half of gestation. *Leptospira bratislava* can localize in the oviduct and uterus of nonpregnant sows and in the genital tract of boars.

The exact way in which *Leptospira* produce their pathogenic effect is not known but capillary damage is a major feature. Localization in the kidney, first in the interstitium and later in the tubules, results in vascular damage and at least temporary damage to tubules. Interstitial nephritis, if extensive, can lead to kidney failure and uremia. The liver may also be affected. In addition, *Leptospira* produce hemolysins which result in the hemolysis of erythrocytes and causes hemoglobinuria and hemolytic anemia.

The severe effects of hemolytic anemia occur mostly in very young piglets. Toxic materials from autolyzing dead fetuses impair the health of the dams and may trigger abortions.

Clinical signs

The acute phase of leptospirosis largely coincides with an initial stage of leptospiremia as well as virulence of the particular serovar involved. Signs often go unnoticed in mature, nonpregnant swine or in growing pigs. A careful observer might notice mild fever and inappetence for a few days. In very young piglets, however, there may be fever, anorexia, hemolytic anemia, hemoglobinuria, icterus, convulsions in occasional pigs and a failure to grow and gain weight.

Chronic infection in dams usually is apparent only as various forms of reproductive failure, including poor conception rates. Pregnant, infected animals often abort in late gestation. In many cases, fetuses are carried almost full term but may be mummified, dead, or weak at birth. Although many infected neonatal pigs die within a few days, some often survive. The dams usually recover promptly. They often conceive again and carry their litters to term.

Lesions

Lesions seldom have been described in sows since most infected adults recover. Grow/finish swine may have scattered foci of interstitial nephritis or generalized kidney scarring which may only be noticed at slaughter as "white-spotted kidneys." Lesions in small piglets include patchy areas of hepatic necrosis, excessive fluid and fibrin in the peritoneal cavity and evidence of inflammation in multiple organs. Microscopically, there is a marked focal, disseminated, interstitial nephritis; tubules and glomeruli often have degeneration and inflammation. Occasionally, a nonsuppurative meningitis can be observed. Placental lesions seldom are marked or significant but may include edema and scattered hemorrhages.

Diagnosis

A history of abortions in late gestation, along with lesions in neonates, may suggest leptospirosis but mere observation is inadequate for accurate diagnosis. Diagnosis of outbreaks is usually based on serologic herd testing. The microscopic agglutination test (MAT), one of several tests available, often is used. Sera from a minimum of 10 animals, including both affected and unaffected animals, should be tested. High antibody titers are usually present at the time of abortion or farrowing but paired samples may be required. Microscopic agglutination testing is serovar specific so the use of multiple assays may be required to arrive at a diagnosis. Breeding animals are commonly vaccinated against multiple *Leptospira* serovars so interpretation of serologic results must also consider vaccination history of the animal. Titers from infection are much higher than those induced by vaccination.

Several other methods of diagnosis sometimes are used but have limitations. These include isolation and identification of leptospires (tedious, laborious), phase contrast identification of leptospires in urine (expensive equipment, not specific), and identification of leptospires in kidney sections with silver stains (lacking sensitivity and specificity). Two rapid and useful techniques, where available, are immunofluorescent microscopy on a homogenate of tissues (kidney, liver, lung, placenta) and immunohistochemistry (IHC). Some laboratories have polymerase chain reaction (PCR) tests that are sensitive but generally not serovar specific.

Control

Control usually is attempted by prevention of exposure, immunization through vaccination, and/or the use of antibiotics. Prevention of exposure is difficult to achieve because so many species can act as carriers of leptospires. These include infected swine, rodents (especially mice and rats) and many kinds of wildlife. Once leptospires are introduced into a favorable wet environment, they often persist there as a source of infection. Nonetheless, leptospirosis can be effectively controlled (perhaps even eradicated) from swine populations raised under confinement conditions using a combination of medication, vaccination, vector control, and providing a treated or non-contaminated drinking water source. Immunization through use of bacterins, widely practiced in breeding herds, usually will reduce the prevalence of infection and abortions. The bacterin must be appropriate for the serovar of *Leptospira* causing the disease. Many bacterins are multivalent. The level of immunity obtained and its duration may not always be satisfactory. Also, bacterins usually will not eliminate infection in carriers. Antibiotics used judiciously may reduce the impact of leptospirosis. It is doubtful that all carriers can be eliminated by the use of permitted antibiotics. Research suggests that oxytetracycline, tylosin, and erythromycin are among the most effective agents.

Mycoplasmal Pneumonia (Enzootic Pneumonia)

Definition

A widespread, chronic respiratory disease of swine characterized by coughing, growth retardation and reduced feed efficiency.

Occurrence

Mycoplasmal pneumonia of swine (MPS, also referred to as "enzootic pneumonia," EP) is a common, widely distributed disease that occurs throughout the year. It is restricted to swine and occurs in all major swine-raising countries. MPS often is more apparent in chronic form on premises where there is continuous flow production and management, and where husbandry and environmental conditions are poor. MPS may cause fairly acute and severe disease in immunologically naïve pigs in age-segregated systems. It may affect pigs early after weaning, when passive immunity has waned, but more commonly occurs in grower and finisher (80-200 lbs) stages. Mycoplasmal pneumonia often interacts with and contributes to other respiratory diseases and is considered to have a central role in porcine respiratory disease complex (PRDC). Secondary bacterial infections are common.

Historical information

Chronic pneumonia in swine, part of which probably was MPS, has been recognized for about a century. MPS was once believed to be caused by a virus and was misnamed "virus pig pneumonia." Clear separation of MPS from swine influenza and recognition of it as a specific disease began in 1948. MPS was first reproduced experimentally in the United States and England in 1965. Subsequently, it was reported in most major swine-raising countries. MPS is now recognized as a very costly, widespread disease of swine, largely because of its negative effects on growth rate and feed efficiency, and its role in PRDC.

Etiology

Mycoplasma hyopneumoniae, the etiologic agent, is difficult to isolate and grows slowly in the laboratory. It is small, filterable, survives only a short time in swine housing environments and can be destroyed by most disinfectants. *Mycoplasma hyopneumoniae* is frequently found in association with other respiratory pathogens, including viruses and bacteria, and is then sometimes termed "porcine respiratory disease complex" (PRDC). In pigs with pneumonia, it may be difficult to determine which agent is the primary pathogen. Evidence suggests that *M. hyopneumoniae* increases the severity of several other infections, including porcine reproductive and respiratory syndrome (PRRS) and influenza, and is capable of acting as a significant primary pathogen on its own.

Two other pathogenic mycoplasmas are recognized in swine. *Mycoplasma hyosynoviae* is a sporadic cause of epidemic synovitis in growing swine. *Mycoplasma hyorhinis* infection is common in swine and it is reported to cause fibrinous polyserositis in young pigs but actual disease attributable to this agent is sporadic.

Epidemiology

Carrier swine are the most common source of infection. Since *M. hyopneumoniae* does not survive for long in the environment, carriers are essential for its maintenance in populations. The organism persists for months in the lungs of infected pigs, including young breeding stock. There is no evidence to implicate infection or carriage in other species. Pigs are infected by *M. hyopneumoniae* transmitted from dams, cohorts, or exposure to other, usually older, pigs. The organism can be frequently isolated from nasal secretions so transmission by nose-to-nose contact and coughing are likely. The organisms also appears to be transmitted by aerosol; empirical evidence suggests that aerosol spread can occur over several miles. A mycoplasma-free status of a herd can be difficult to maintain.

Pathogenesis

Mycoplasma hyopneumoniae can be observed microscopically on ciliary epithelium of trachea, bronchi and bronchioles. Distribution of pulmonary lesions suggests bronchogenic distribution with settling of exudate cranioventrally because of compromised mucociliary apparatus. Virulence factors derived from *M. hyopneumoniae* outer membrane proteins damage several respiratory defense mechanisms and facilitate infection. The cell membrane presents a mosaic of epitopes that camouflage protective antigens, rendering immune response inefficient. Poor air quality (dust or noxious gases) can irritate airways and increase susceptibility.

The initial lesions are bronchitis and bronchiolitis. There is hyperplasia of mucus secreting cells in the mucosa and a loss of cilia from many epithelial cells of airways. The inflammatory reaction spreads into surrounding alveoli causing alveolitis, pneumonia, airway obstruction, and atelectasis. Over time there is a marked hyperplasia of lymphoid tissue around airways and adjacent blood vessels. Increased mucus in airways, ciliostasis, and pressure of surrounding lymphoid tissue interfere with the lung clearance of mucus and exudate. Secondary bacterial infections contribute substantially and are the usual cause of severe pneumonia and deaths.

Clinical signs

The principal clinical sign is chronic, persistent, nonproductive cough. Onset often occurs about two to three weeks after exposure and usually is gradual in a herd. Coughing may persist for weeks to months. Excessive dust, irritating gases, or concurrent infections result in more severe coughing. As pneumonia develops in some pigs, dyspnea becomes more marked. Growth is retarded and feed efficiency decreases in the face of near-normal appetites. Morbidity is high and mortality is low.

Lesions

In affected pigs, pneumonic lesions are predominantly well demarcated and cranioventral, involving apical, intermediate, and cardiac lobes but extend into diaphragmatic lobes in severe cases. Chronic lesions usually are reduced in volume (atelectic) and dark gray. More recent lesions tend to be reddish brown or a lighter gray, with edema, mucus, and inflammatory cells apparent in the airways. Raised areas adjacent to pneumonic areas often are emphysematous and lighter pink than normal lung. On cut surface of pneumonic areas, mucopurulent exudate often can be squeezed from airways. Secondary infection with other respiratory pathogens is common and may modify the appearance of mycoplasma-initiated lesions.

Typical microscopic lesions, although not pathognomonic, reveal lymphohistiocytic peribronchiolar cuffing, mucocellular exudates, and atelectasis.

Neither gross nor microscopic lesions are pathognomonic for *M. hyopneumoniae*. Cranioventral or bronchogenic, clearly demarcated consolidation of lungs is a characteristic of bacterial bronchopneumonia and is not always associated with the presence of *M. hyopneumoniae*.

Diagnosis

History, signs, gross and microscopic lesions are suggestive of *M. hyopneumoniae* but laboratory assistance is needed for accurate diagnostic confirmation. Isolation is slow, laborious, difficult and generally not routinely available. Identification of the agent in lung samples taken at necropsy is possible using fluorescent antibody, immunohistochemical, or polymerase chain reaction (PCR) techniques. Serologic tests including complement fixation and enzyme-linked immunosorbent assay (ELISA) tests can be useful on a herd basis but interpretation must be made with care and knowledge of the herd, individuals sampled, and vaccination status.

Tests on individual animals have little value because many pigs without active disease have antibodies to *M. hyopneumoniae* or other cross-reacting mycoplasmas. Antibody levels develop slowly in many infected animals. A recently developed, nested PCR test on nasal or lung swabs collected from live pigs permits earlier, more accurate diagnosis of infection. Detection of the organism by PCR confirms the presence of the organism but does not confirm its role in disease.

A careful study of lung lesions at slaughter by one familiar with gross lesions of MPS can be of value in determining prevalence and evaluating progress toward control. However, many gross lesions heal by the time that pigs reach market weight and other bacterial pneumonias may mimic the gross lesions of *M. hyopneumoniae*. For differential diagnosis, see the table, Respiratory Diseases, on page 159.

Control

Many methods of control are in use and many herds supplying genetic stock are maintained negative for *M. hyopneumoniae*. Such herds obviously must have scrupulous isolation, acclimatization, testing, and biosecurity protocols in place to assure the organism is not introduced with breeding stock.

Most negative herds are the result of depopulation and repopulation with negative breeding stock. In some cases, herds have become negative through strict medicated or segregated early weaning, and other minimal disease programs. Specific pathogen free (SPF) herds are derived from pigs taken via hysterectomy or cesarean section and raised on colostrum-free diets. They are then used to repopulate clean, swine-raising facilities. Maintaining commercial herds free of *M. hyopneumoniae* infection when located in swine-dense regions has not been successful long term. A control strategy developed in Europe and referred to as "Swiss depopulation" has gained favor in recent years. The technique is based on a hypothesis that most adult swine raised on an endemically infected farm are exposed to *M. hyopneumoniae* early in life with subsequent recovery (and presumably robust immunity with limited carrier status) by 10 months of age. Swiss depopulation involves a period of intensive vaccination of all breeding animals on a farm followed by removal of all animals less than 10 months of age. For a period of approximately three-weeks following this, on-site farrowing is stopped. During the stand-down period, all animals remaining on the farm are intensively treated with antibiotics aimed at elimination of any *M. hyopneumoniae* organisms that may be residing in carrier animals. Removal of all susceptible swine combined with vaccination/medication programs generally results in a significant decrease in effect from the disease for up to two years with eradication of the organism reported in some instances.

Other measures to aid in control but not elimination include early weaning, medicated early weaning (MEW) or modifications of MEW. Piglets are weaned before 21 days of age. Early weaning may prevent transmission of *M. hyopneumoniae* (and other organisms) from dams to piglets before they are weaned and moved to a separate, clean nursery or grow/finish facility. Age segregated rearing and the all in/all out system of management with cleaning and disinfection of facilities between batches of pigs is widely used and believed to be one of the more practical and useful measures.

Despite methods to eliminate or control *M. hyopneumoniae*, it remains a significant economic problem, particularly when PRRS virus or swine influenza virus (SIV) is endemic. Vaccines are generally thought to be efficacious and can be effective in mitigating losses due to *M. hyopneumoniae* infection. Vaccines reduce lung lesions and improve growth performance. In some systems, sows are vaccinated once or twice several weeks before farrowing but most programs rely on vaccination of piglets. In most herds, maternal antibodies do not seem to interfere with piglet vaccination. Piglets are usually vaccinated before weaning and again two to three weeks later.

Antibiotics may augment management and vaccination techniques and can be given in feed, water, or by injection. Many antibiotics and chemotherapeutic agents have been used in feed or water for prevention or treatment, often with inconsistent results. Efficacy of antimicrobials in controlling *M. hyopneumoniae* losses may be related either to antimycoplasmal activity or suppression of other infections. Those reported efficacious specifically for *M. hyopneumoniae* include lincomycin, tiamulin, tetracyclines, tylosin, tilmicosin, tulathromycin, enrofloxacin and perhaps others.

Pneumonic Pasteurellosis (Pasteurellosis; *Pasteurella multocida*; also see Atrophic Rhinitis)

Definition

This disease of swine is usually seen in association with other infectious diseases or environmental factors that impair pulmonary function. There are both primary and secondary forms of the disease.

Occurrence

Pneumonic pasteurellosis (PP) occurs throughout the world. Secondary PP is seen in association with several other diseases, especially mycoplasmal pneumonia, viral infections of lung, and *Actinobacillus pleuropneumoniae*. It often accompanies or follows unusual environmental or other stresses. Similar forms of pasteurellosis occur in many other species, including cattle (genus renamed *Mannheimia*), rabbits, fowl, sheep and rodents.

Primary pasteurellosis occurs occasionally as a septicemic disease with meningitis in piglets. A septicemic form also occurs rarely in older or adult swine. Secondary pasteurellosis is seen much more frequently than primary pasteurellosis.

Historical information

In the early days of bacteriology, Pasteur experimented with a disease of poultry now believed to have been fowl cholera caused by *Pasteurella multocida;* the genus, *Pasteurella*, was named after him. Subsequent research implicated *Pasteurella multocida* as an important primary and secondary pathogen in many species, including swine.

Etiology

The etiologic agent is *Pasteurella multocida*, a Gram-negative coccobacillus easily grown in the laboratory. There are both toxigenic and non-toxigenic strains. The organism is a common inhabitant of the pig's nasal passages and can be isolated from most swine herds. There are five capsular serotypes (A, B, D, E, and F) and 16 somatic serotypes. In the United States, pneumonic pasteurellosis of swine is caused by serotypes A and D.

Epidemiology

Carrier swine probably introduce *P. multocida* into most herds, with subsequent vertical and lateral transmission. Transmission is suspected of being via nose-to-nose contact. Although many other species harbor *P. multocida*; there is little evidence of interspecies transfer of strains pathogenic for swine.

Pathogenesis

Healthy swine are highly resistant to experimental infection by *P. multocida* and many normal swine are carriers of *P. multocida* in their nasopharynx. Chronic, progressive pneumonia occurs when resistance has been lowered and the organism colonizes deeper portions of the lung.

Pathogenic strains appear to produce their effect largely through damage to microvasculature in the lung. This leads to the formation of fibrinous thrombi in alveolar capillaries and escape of fibrinogen into alveoli where it is converted to fibrin. The fibrin then can be slowly organized into fibrous connective tissue. Abscesses that may develop in the pneumonic lung may be a consequence of infarction of localized areas or the result of a necrotizing effect of toxic products produced by *P. multocida* and other secondary bacteria.

The severe inflammatory reaction that accompanies the process sometimes involves pleura and occasionally the pericardial sac. Fibrin on the pleura overlying pneumonic lesions may organize to form fibrous adhesions that attach the lung to the rib cage, but this finding is more often due to prior effects of *Actinobacillus*, *Haemophilus*, or *Streptococcus* infection. Since the agent is common, easily isolated, and persists in lesions, *P. multocida* is frequently isolated from lungs in which there are other primary agents of pneumonia (*Actinobacillus sp.*, swine influenza, *Mycoplasma hyopneumoniae*). In acute cases, bacteremia and septicemia can occur and deaths are believed to be caused by endotoxic shock and respiratory failure.

Clinical signs

Signs vary in severity and are those often seen with other types of pneumonia: coughing, dyspnea, fever and prostration. Chronic cases tend to have less fever, a persistent cough and a more marked dyspnea. Swine with well-developed pneumonia or extensive adhesions between lungs and rib cage often have a marked expiratory lift ("thump").

Lesions

Pneumonic areas involve the cranioventral lobes of the lungs and often extend to adjacent parts of the diaphragmatic lobes. Pneumonic areas are remarkable for their firmness and density. The pleura over lesion areas may be granular and scant fibrin may be visible on the surface. Regional lymph nodes usually are enlarged. Microscopic lesions are those of a suppurative bronchopneumonia. Fibrin and bacteria often are prominent in affected alveoli and, sometimes, in interalveolar capillaries. Occasionally, acute necrotizing pharyngitis and fibrinous polyarthritis without joint swelling are present. Less often, there is meningitis or meningoencephalitis.

Diagnosis

History, signs and the remarkable pulmonary lesions may be suggestive of pneumonic pasteurellosis but culture of lung lesions from a nonmedicated pig is required for confirmation. Pneumonic pasteurellosis is often secondary to one or more of a host of primary diseases that should not be overlooked. Environmental factors such as dusty or overcrowded conditions, excessive ammonia gas or poor ventilation may be important predisposing factors. Only when all other possible causes have been eliminated should there be a diagnosis of primary PP.

Serology and mere isolation of *P. multocida* from nasal swabs is of little value without being able to predict pathogenicity. The application of the polymerase chain reaction (PCR) to detect and differentiate toxin producing and nontoxin producing *P. multocida* may prove to be a useful technique for control of both pneumonic pasteurellosis and atrophic rhinitis.

Control

Control methods include all the measures that might prevent introduction of a new strain of *P. multocida* into a herd. Herd additions should be quarantined for at least a few weeks. Use of the all in/all out system of raising swine will reduce the likelihood of PP. Mixing and sorting of pigs should be minimized. Implementing control of other respiratory pathogens (e.g. *M. hyopneumoniae*, porcine reproductive and respiratory syndrome virus (PRRSV), swine influenza, *A. pleuropneumoniae*) or any other disease, environmental or stress factor that might lower resistance should be addressed.

Bacterins against *P. multocida* are available but their efficacy in preventing or minimizing the severity of respiratory disease is questionable.

Pneumonic pasteurellosis is difficult to treat effectively. Basic therapeutic caveats of early diagnosis, appropriate choice of antimicrobial, and appropriate dose with sufficient duration of therapy are particularly important for success. Many different antibiotics (tiamulin, tulathromycin, lincomycin with chlortetracycline, penicillins, tilmicosin, tetracyclines, etc) have been recommended for injection or oral medication. In selecting an antimicrobial, it may be useful to run sensitivity tests on the organism isolated from a typical non-treated sick pig in the herd.

Proliferative Enteritis (Porcine Proliferative Enteritis, Ileitis, Intestinal Adenomatosis, Garden-hose Gut)

Definition

Porcine proliferative enteritis (PPE) is an enteric disease characterized by hyperplasia of crypt enterocytes with inflammation and sometimes ulceration or hemorrhage. Lesions always include thickening of the mucous membrane of part of the small intestine and/or large intestine. Lesions vary considerably by location, extent, and duration. Many terms have been used to describe this disease, including: proliferative hemorrhagic enteropathy (PHE), porcine intestinal adenomatosis (PIA), porcine proliferative enteritis (PPE), necrotic enteritis (NE), regional or terminal ileitis (RI), ileitis, and garden-hose gut.

Occurrence

Porcine proliferative enteritis (PPE) occurs worldwide. Disease is categorized pathologically as a severe acute form (proliferative hemorrhagic enteropathy or PHE) that is more common in young adults, and a chronic or necrotic form which occurs much more frequently, usually during the grower phase.

The disease occurs primarily in growing/finishing pigs but may also occur in pigs as young as 3 weeks, in market weight hogs and adult swine. Disease often appears to be more severe with, and occurs at an increased incidence in, age-segregated herds. Similar signs and lesions occur in other mammals (hamsters, ferrets, guinea pigs, foxes, horses, lambs, rabbits, rats, dogs, white-tailed deer, emus) with no detectable differences in the genotype of the causative organism. Hamsters have been used in research and are readily infected by the porcine organism.

Historical information

The first report of PPE was published in 1931. Neither that nor another report in 1935 stimulated much interest. In the 1970s there was a renewed interest as marked losses from PPE became more apparent. In 1993, a method of cultivation of the confirmed etiologic agent (*Lawsonia intracellularis*) in tissue culture was reported. The agent has now been used to reproduce the disease in conventional, susceptible pigs.

Etiology

Bent, rod-shaped, Gram-negative bacteria in crypt enterocytes of swine with PPE were recognized long ago. However, the organism could not be grown on cell-free media and was not identified until 1993. The obligate intracellular organism, *Lawsonia intracellularis* (Li) is considered to be a novel taxonomic genus and species. It is related to certain anaerobic, sulfate-reducing bacteria.

Lawsonia intracellularis can be grown in a rat enterocyte cell line and inoculation of susceptible pigs with pure culture of the organism reproduces PPE. All isolates examined from different host species and from different geographical locations appear to be quite similar. Polymerase chain reaction (PCR) has been useful for characterization of the organism and has ruled-out involvement of *Campylobacter spp.* in the disease

Epidemiology

The incubation, recovery, and carrier phase of *L. intracellularis* infection is quite long in some pigs, probably months. Undoubtedly, there are carrier swine that disseminate *L. intracellularis* in their feces to susceptible pigs by fecal-oral route. Infection often results in subclinical disease. Research also shows that *L. intracellularis* from experimentally infected pigs spreads to naive sentinel pigs penned with them or penned separately in the same enclosed area.

Carrier dams have been demonstrated to infect their litters as early as six days of age, a likely reason for failure of segregated early weaning techniques to control disease. The incubation period is at least two weeks, perhaps much longer. Outbreaks often have been associated with a variety of stresses. Lateral transmission of infection has been demonstrated but not all pigs within a population are necessarily infected simultaneously.

Pathogenesis

L. intracellularis infects epithelial cells and survives intracellularly. When enterocytes undergo mitosis, each cell retains some of the bacteria, and enterocytes fail to mature. The resulting hallmark lesion is a proliferation of immature enterocytes. Whether the organism stimulates greater proliferation, retards maturation, or both is not known. Microscopically, organisms are visible within the apex of crypt epithelial cells. Responses to the bacteria include crypt elongation, epithelial cell hyperplasia, degeneration and necrosis of enterocytes, fewer goblet cells, and an inflammatory response.

Other details of pathogenesis are speculative. Variations in the reported syndromes may correlate with different stages in lesion development or different responses to infection, perhaps modulated by predisposing factors, stresses and saprophytic organisms. Seroconversion occurs two weeks after infection, although lesions may not develop for three to four weeks post-infection. The protected, intracellular environment afforded the organism probably requires a cell-mediated response to eliminate infection. Resolution of lesions starts approximately four weeks after infection.

Clinical signs

There has been much confusion related to nomenclature, lesions, and clinical signs of PPE, primarily due to the variation that exists in clinical signs, age of pig affected, and gross lesions. In addition, a syndrome (hemorrhagic bowel syndrome or HBS) of sudden death with blood in the intestinal tract (which is not PPE) is often confused with this condition. Acute cases of PPE are most frequently observed in late finishing pigs and young breeding stock (PHE). Acute diarrhea with brownish to black unclotted blood, pallor, weakness, and rapid death are common; lesions include mucosal proliferation and hemorrhage. Subacute to chronic cases occur more frequently in the grower stages, manifested by sporadic diarrhea, wasting, and variation in growth rate; lesions often include necrotic enteritis and can be easily confused with salmonellosis. Morbidity and mortality with either presentation is variable. Some pigs may have quite severe proliferation of mucosa of terminal small intestine yet can be clinically asymptomatic.

Lesions

Lesions vary in severity and location but usually include gross thickening of some part of the mucosa of the small and/or large intestine. The ileum is commonly affected, often with a hose-like thickening of the mucosa of terminal ileum. A cerebriform pattern (resembling the external fissures and convolution of the brain) of intestinal thickening is visible from serosal surface. Peyer's patches may be hyperplastic. Bloody intestinal content, perhaps with frank blood clots, may be present, especially in PHE. Lesions occasionally are present only in the large intestine. In these instances, the mucosa of the cecum and/or colon is thrown into thick folds, plaques or polyps, may be covered by inflammatory exudate, and vaguely resembles lesions of swine dysentery, trichuriasis, or salmonellosis. Healing lesions of PPE in many slaughtered hogs suggest that some affected swine may show few or no signs and recover spontaneously.

In conventionally stained histologic sections there is severe intestinal crypt cell hyperplasia; in silver stained sections or with immunohistochemistry, curved to rod-shaped bacteria usually can be demonstrated in the apex of some enterocytes.

Diagnosis

A tentative diagnosis often can be made on the basis of clinical signs along with the presence of characteristic gross and microscopic lesions, although some cases of porcine circovirus type 2 (PCV2) enteritis can present themselves clinically very similar to PPE. Laboratories use silver stains, immunohistochemistry, or fluorescent antibody tests on histologic sections to confirm the presence of the organism within lesions. Polymerase chain reaction (PCR) testing on samples of affected mucosa or feces is also available. PCR performed on feces from clinically affected pigs is diagnostic but negative tests do not rule out carrier status. Serology has limited availability and unknown sensitivity. Antibody specific for *L. intracellularis* appears to have low magnitude and duration but testing can be useful on a herd basis to determine if the herd is infected and when infection may be occurring.

Control

Prevention by elimination is difficult; segregated rearing has been largely unsuccessful. There is no certainty that exposure of swine to *L. intracellularis* can be avoided. More information is needed on survival of the organism under field conditions and the role other animals may play in transmission and/or reservoirs. Presently there is no widely available way to screen large numbers of apparently normal, suspected carriers. Serologic tests eventually may be useful for identifying infected herds. Although PCR is not yet widely available, it can identify *Lawsonia intracellularis* in fecal samples from clinically affected pigs but lacks sensitivity to identify inapparent carriers.

Outbreaks sometimes appear to be stress related. Environmental and other stresses, including transportation, sorting, or commingling, often precipitate outbreaks and should be minimized.

Various antibiotics often are added to feed for several weeks during or after periods of stress and during outbreaks in order to control and treat PPE. Experimental PPE can be controlled using tylosin, tetracyclines, lincomycin, tiamulin, and carbadox. Various medication strategies have been used, including pulse dosing and continuous medication. Medication failures are common in breeding stock where animals are not fed ad libitum, hence receive subtherapeutic doses of antimicrobials that might otherwise be effective. Control of PPE has been a major reason for use of feed-grade antimicrobials in grow-finish swine.

An avirulent live vaccine is widely available and appears to have very good efficacy when properly administered via water or orally. Vaccination of growing pigs as well as breeding gilts during acclimatization has been very successful in reducing or eliminating clinical signs of PPE. In some herds, vaccination has allowed the elimination of continuous administration of feed-grade antimicrobials.

Salmonellosis

Definition

Salmonellosis is the disease caused by any of more than 2000 *Salmonella* serotypes. In swine, only a few serotypes cause disease, usually manifested as septicemia and/or enterocolitis, sometimes by tissue localization of infection at various sites. *Salmonella* infections in asymptomatic swine may serve as a source of *Salmonella* infection to humans via contamination of pork products.

Occurrence

Infection of swine with a broad range of serotypes is common. Disease as a result of infection is relatively less common but occurs throughout the year in all major swine-raising countries. All age groups are susceptible but the disease usually occurs in weaned or growing/finishing pigs. Many other species, including people, are susceptible to salmonellosis caused by some of the *Salmonella* serotypes that affect swine. Contaminated pork products are not a primary source of food-borne salmonellosis outbreaks in people but efforts to reduce salmonellae in the pork food chain are a high priority for the swine industry.

Historical information

In 1886 the organism now known as *Salmonella* serotype Choleraesuis was erroneously reported to cause hog cholera. After the viral etiology for hog cholera was identified, salmonellae were thought of as secondary pathogens. However *Salmonella* serotypes frequently do act as primary pathogens causing septicemia and/or enterocolitis in swine.

It has been shown that some outbreaks of salmonellosis in people are food-borne and that food products of animal origin, including pork, are sometimes are implicated as the source of these outbreaks. Species-adapted *Salmonella* serotypes are relatively infrequent; most serotypes are capable of infecting (though not necessarily causing disease in) multiple mammalian hosts. Both animal and human health could be improved if salmonellosis could be effectively controlled across animal production and food processing systems. *Salmonella* reduction programs at farm level constitute a logical step in minimizing the occurrence of outbreaks in humans. Swine industry-led national *Salmonella* control programs in North America and Europe are being implemented in an effort to understand what management strategies are most likely to minimize the impact of the organism on both human and animal health.

Etiology

Salmonella is now recognized as a genus with about 2000 serotypes that can be serologically clustered in groups (see serogroup examples in Table 1). Pathogenic serotypes for swine are relatively few, with most outbreaks caused by *Salmonella* Choleraesuis or *Salmonella* serotype Typhimurium. Serotypes that are the most common cause of disease in both people and swine include *Salmonella* serotypes Typhimurium, Enteritidis, Agona and Heidelberg. *Salmonella* Choleraesuis and *Salmonella* serotype Typhisuis are host-adapted to swine and are rarely isolated from sources other than infected swine.

Salmonellae are small, hardy, ubiquitous, Gram-negative bacilli. All contain endotoxin and are capable of elaborating a variety of other toxins. They can readily survive in many swine environments but can be inactivated by chlorine, iodine and phenol-based disinfectants.

Epidemiology

Asymptomatic, clinically normal swine may harbor inapparent *Salmonella* infections that persist in their tonsils, intestine, lymph nodes, or gall bladder. Those carrier swine regularly or occasionally shed salmonellae in their feces and present a major source of exposure to susceptible swine. Mingling of healthy pigs with sick or inapparent carriers often precipitates an outbreak of salmonellosis. Once introduced, salmonellae are spread by the fecal-oral

Table 1: Common serotypes of *Salmonella enterica* serogroups B, C1, C2, D and E isolated from US pigs

Group B	Group C1	Group C2	Group D	Group E
Abortus-equi	Choleraesuis	Hadar	Dublin	Anatum
Agona	Infantis	Kentucky	Enteritidis	Meleagridis
Brandenburg	Lille	Litchfield	Miami	Muenster
Bredeney	Mbandaka	Manhattan		New Brunswick
California	Montevideo	Muechen		Orien
Derby	Tennessee	Newport		Riefild
Heidelberg	Thompson			Senftenberg
Saint Paul				Uganda
San Diego				
Schwarzengrund				
Typhimurium				

route, in contaminated feed and water, or sometimes by aerosol. Exposed pigs may either develop clinical signs of salmonellosis or resist infection and remain healthy. Any pig exposed to salmonellae should subsequently be considered as a possible carrier of the organism.

Contaminated buildings and pens remain infectious for weeks and pigs moved into them are likely to become infected. Historically, feed was a major source of new infections and remains so for many serotypes. *Salmonella* Choleraesuis, a host-adapted and frequent cause of disease in swine, has never been reported as a feed contaminant. Most serotypes are capable of infecting a broad host range. For example, *S.* Typhimurium frequently infects many other kinds of animals, including livestock, poultry and mice, is readily transmitted between species, and occasionally is found in feedstuffs. Rodents and wild birds are believed to be important disseminators of *Salmonella* organisms.

Salmonellosis often appears during or following stressful events, e.g. prolonged transport, drought, overcrowding, change of rations, parturition, prolonged treatment with drugs or antibiotics, or another disease in the herd. Unusual stress lowers resistance and/or increases magnitude of shedding, hence dose, and can precipitate outbreaks. A balance of virulence, dose, and resistance exists between swine and the salmonellae they carry or with which they become infected.

Pathogenesis

Following ingestion or inhalation of *S.* Choleraesuis, the organisms invade tonsil and/or intestinal mucosa and soon spread to regional lymph nodes, usually with septicemia. Other *Salmonella* serotypes usually remain confined to the intestine and, perhaps, adjacent lymph nodes producing only a transient septicemia. Host-adapted *S.* Choleraesuis, and occasionally other serotypes, sometimes are phagocytized and survive within macrophages and neutrophils that transport them to other sites where they localize and cause lesions. Sites include lungs, liver, brain, meninges, joints and lymph nodes.

In enteric salmonellosis as typified by infection with *S.* Typhimurium, mucosal damage and necrosis are the result of mucosal ischemia caused by vasculitis and microvascular thrombosis. Vasculitis is present in all forms of salmonellosis. Diarrhea is attributed to tissue fluids leaking from damaged mucosa and compromise of mucosal absorption. An enterotoxin similar to that produced by enterotoxigenic *E. coli* (causing cyclic AMP-mediated hypersecretion of fluids and salts from enterocytes) has been described for *Salmonella* Heidelberg.

Clinical signs

Septicemic salmonellosis usually is caused by host adapted *Salmonella* Choleraesuis. It usually is seen in pigs from weaning to about 180 pounds but can occur in all ages of swine. Lactogenic immunity is usually protective. Acute onset of an outbreak may be signaled by acute death loss in a group of apparently thrifty pigs. Within a few days the disease spreads among other pigs in the group. Morbidity usually is low to moderate but mortality is high among those that become ill.

Clinical signs include inappetence, depression, huddling, weakness, temperatures up to 107° F (41.6° C), and red to purple discoloration of skin of the extremities (cyanosis). Diarrhea is not present initially but occurs after a few days of illness. The length of course is variable, both in individual animals and in the herd and may be influenced by treatment.

The enterocolitic form of salmonellosis usually is caused by *Salmonella* Typhimurium and less often by *S.* Choleraesuis or other serotypes. This form tends to involve pigs from weaning to about 180 pounds. Initial signs include moderate anorexia and diarrhea that may be watery to yellow and intermittent. Animals are moderately febrile initially but temperatures usually regress as diarrhea continues. As the disease progresses, there may be mucus, fibrin, and blood in the feces but blood is not a prominent feature. Over time, morbidity is high and mortality is moderate. Surviving animals often become emaciated or gain weight slowly.

Localization of salmonellae sometimes occurs in the lungs, brain, meninges and lymph nodes. Less common sites include gall bladder, joints and synovium. Localization in the lungs can lead to cough or dyspnea, or in the brain to central nervous system (CNS) signs.

Lesions

In septicemic salmonellosis, gross lesions include red to purplish discoloration of the extremities, marked enlargement of the spleen, moderate swelling of the liver, swollen and wet lymph nodes and reddening of the fundic part of the stomach. Frequently there will be petechial hemorrhages in skin, larynx, lungs, heart, bladder and kidneys. The liver may or may not contain small, white to yellow foci of necrosis (paratyphoid nodules). In animals with localization of infection in the lungs, there is pulmonary congestion and edema and patchy consolidation; in the brain or meninges, congestion and, perhaps, hemorrhages; in joints, villous proliferation.

Intestinal lesions vary in severity, largely related to duration of illness. At onset there may be only congestion with superficial fibrinous inflammation of small or large areas of the cecum, colon and terminal end of the small intestine. In long standing cases the intestinal lesions resemble those of the enterocolitic form of salmonellosis.

In the enterocolitic form of salmonellosis, the large intestine and the lower small intestine are heavy, edematous and the wall is thickened. There may be excessive peritoneal fluid and strands of fibrin on the serosa. Ileocolic and mesenteric lymph nodes usually are markedly enlarged, congested and edematous. There is a marked enterocolitis with focal or diffuse areas of mucosal necrosis with fibrinonecrotic exudates in small intestine, cecum, colon and/or rectum. In chronic cases there may be raised, circular lesions in the colon ("button ulcers"). Rectal stricture with accompanying megacolon has been described as a sequelae to *Salmonella* infection. Dry gangrene may occur on the ears or tail of survivors.

Diagnosis

The history, clinical signs and typical gross lesions may be adequate for a tentative diagnosis. Diagnosis should be confirmed by laboratory culture and identification of *Salmonella*, especially if the disease is new on the premises. Serogrouping is readily available and can aid in determining potential serotypes involved (see Table 1); serotyping is available upon request and is sometimes useful to define epidemiology and expected clinical outcome. A few typical, untreated animals, preferably alive, should be submitted for culture and histopathologic study. Diagnosticians often culture multiple organs including liver, spleen, lung, mesenteric lymph nodes and colon. Microscopic examination of tissues will help identify typical lesions and differentiate them from those of other enteric and septicemic diseases. *Salmonella* Choleraesuis typically causes rather unique paratyphoid nodules in the liver.

Septicemic salmonellosis must be differentiated carefully from classical swine fever, erysipelas and other septicemias as well as other causes of interstitial pneumonia. The enterocolitic form must be differentiated from coliform enteritis, porcine proliferative enteritis, trichuriasis, and swine dysentery. The latter two diseases tend to be restricted to the large intestine.

Control

Breeding stock should be acquired only from suppliers with no recent history of salmonellosis. If feasible, all breeding stock should be from a single source. Essential additions to the herd should be made only after a quarantine period of 30-60 days.

Ideally, only pigs from a single source and of similar age should be raised together in a closed, all in/all out system. Buildings should be cleaned and disinfected carefully between batches. All possible carriers, including rodents, birds, pets and wildlife, should be eradicated or excluded. Unusual stresses should be avoided insofar as possible. Perhaps the most important approach to control of salmonellosis involves comfortable dry housing, proper animal density, good ventilation and a high standard of sanitation. Early weaning and removal of piglets to a separate, clean site has been successful in avoiding transmission of *S.* Choleraesuis from breeding populations known to include carriers.

For control of *Salmonella* Choleraesuis, and perhaps *S.* Typhimurium, avirulent live vaccines are available and quite effective. Killed *Salmonella* bacterins and a mutant-derived endotoxin vaccine are available but thought to be less effective. All vaccination programs should be coupled with proper sanitation, husbandry and pig flow.

Numerous antibiotics and chemotherapeutic agents have been used for prevention and/or treatment. Some reduce mortality as well as the duration and severity of salmonellosis. Frequently used products include carbadox, gentamycin, neomycin, tiamulin, ceftiofur, and others. Systemically absorbed or injectable antimicrobials are preferred for septicemic salmonellosis. Because salmonellae have developed resistance to many therapeutic agents, isolation and antimicrobial sensitivity are usually warranted. It has not been confirmed that treatment of infected pigs with antimicrobials induces a *Salmonella* carrier status as has been suggested in humans.

Successful reduction of salmonella infections in swine herds has been reported in Europe and the US. The programs are based largely on serologic testing of breeding stock, culture of samples taken at slaughter, establishment of measures that reduce contamination of carcasses at slaughter, and controlling risks that are likely to result in introduction of *Salmonella* through feed or drinking water. The hazard analysis critical control point (HACCP) programs instituted by United States abattoirs have adopted many of these measures.

Streptococcal Infections

The predominant streptococcal disease of swine is caused by *Streptococcus suis*. Other less common, largely sporadic, streptococcal infections are summarized as follows.

Sporadic infections occasionally are caused by *Streptococcus equisimilis*. This beta-hemolytic streptococcus and a few others sometimes cause arthritis, septicemia or meningitis in young pigs, complicate other disease processes, or may contribute to cases of vegetative, valvular endocarditis in older growing/finishing pigs. This organism is indigenous in the vagina and infects pigs at birth. The cases in young pigs are a result of navel infection or from breaks in the integument as a result of knee abrasions, or infection of skin wounds including those caused by tail docking, ear notching or clipping of needle teeth.

Streptococcus porcinus is the same as Lancefield group E streptococci associated with jowl abscess (feeder boils) in swine. This disease was once quite prevalent but is now rare, presumably because of improvements in husbandry and feeder design. It is occasionally isolated from pigs with septicemia or abscesses.

Additional streptococci believed to be pathogens have been isolated from the respiratory tract, mammary glands, localized skin lesions and subcutaneous abscesses, from the reproductive tract of aborting sows, and sows with fertility problems or agalactia. Their role in these conditions is less clear. *Streptococcus durans* has been associated with enteritis in suckling pigs.

Streptococcus suis Infection

Definition

This is the most important streptococcal infection of pigs and is usually seen in nursing or recently weaned piglets. The disease usually is characterized by septicemia, acute meningitis, polyarthritis, polyserositis, or bronchopneumonia.

Occurrence

Although *S. suis* infection occurs primarily in nursing or recently weaned pigs, all age groups occasionally are affected. The disease is found in all major swine-raising countries. It is relatively common, occurs throughout the year, and is prevalent in confinement-raised swine. *Streptococcus suis* infection also occurs sporadically in several domestic animals (cattle, sheep, goats, horses, dogs). It is zoonotic and occurs occasionally in people who work with pigs or handle meats (butchers, farmers, and veterinarians), causing localized infections, arthritis, septicemia and possibly death.

Historical information

Outbreaks of streptococcal infection in swine occurred many years before the organism, *S. suis*, was identified in 1987 as a new pathogenic species. Outbreaks of *S. suis* infection now are reported frequently. Because *S. suis* colonizes piglets at birth, both segregated early weaning (SEW) and medicated early weaning (MEW) fail to prevent *S. suis* infections.

There has been much research on streptococci. Early research on *S. suis* largely concerned capsular serotypes and comparison of signs and lesions produced by different serotypes. Virulence factors have been the focus of more recent research. Infection models vary widely and likely contribute to the lack of agreement in findings reported in published studies.

Etiology

Streptococcus suis is Gram-positive and easily grown on blood agar. Identification is based on biochemical reactions and capsular serotyping. There are about 35 capsular serotypes. Their prevalence varies in different geographic regions of the US with types 2, 3, 4 and 7 predominating in the Midwest. Type 2 may be most prevalent worldwide and is the most likely to express virulence. Virulence factors are not well understood but capsular polysaccharide (CPS) and two proteins, muramidase released protein (MRP) and an extracellular factor (EF) are thought to play important roles in the severity of disease caused by infection with type 2.

Many species of *Streptococcus* can be isolated from normal swine. There is no single, consistent predictor of possible pathogenicity. Environmental or other predisposing factors may influence pathogenicity. Most streptococci are readily destroyed by common disinfectants such as phenol, quaternary ammonium, formaldehyde, hypochlorite, chlorhexidine, or 3% iodine.

Epidemiology

Streptococcus suis survives in dust and feces in the usual swine environment. It can be isolated from the nasal cavity and palatine tonsils of many normal pigs. It is present in the feces and nasal secretions of carriers. Transmission may be through ingestion, inhalation or nose-to-nose contact. Flies and rodents may play a role in mechanical spread. *S. suis* can survive on flies for at least 5 days.

Healthy carrier swine usually introduce infection. Sows infect piglets at or shortly after birth. Contaminated secretions, excretions and skin of infected pigs also expose other pigs. These factors may make early weaning (7-24 days) and MEW ineffective in preventing transmission to at least some piglets which may then serve as sources of infection to cohorts during lactation and nursery phases. Wounds also are a common route of entry for *S. suis*. Once a few piglets are infected, they are able to disseminate the bacteria to other litters or commingled pigs. Close contact favors spread.

Multiple serotypes may exist on the same farm. Control of a particular type of *S. suis* may lead to emergence of another serotype, frustrating long-term control strategies.

Pathogenesis

Pathogenesis is somewhat speculative and may differ among different serotypes. Management and husbandry stresses may predispose piglets to outbreaks. Also, preexisting injury to respiratory epithelium, especially rhinitis, may predispose to infection. Known causes of rhinitis include ammonia fumes, infection with *Bordetella bronchiseptica* and *Pasteurella multocida*, and inclusion body rhinitis. Interaction of *S. suis* with viruses (pseudorabies, swine influenza, porcine reproductive and respiratory syndrome [PRRS]) may trigger some outbreaks.

After oral or respiratory entry, streptococci pass to the crypts of the palatine tonsils. From there the organisms invade via lymphatics to the mandibular lymph nodes where they can remain localized or become septicemic. Some organisms may survive within phagocytes and gain access to cerebrospinal fluid, brain, meninges, lungs and joints where they localize and cause meningoencephalitis, arthritis or pneumonia. In pneumonic lungs, *S. suis* can be either a primary or secondary pathogen.

Clinical signs

Signs and lesions are similar in all *S. suis* infections, regardless of serotype. Signs usually suggest septicemia and/or localization of systemic infection. Pigs with septicemia die after a short, acute course and may not have been observed as sick pigs. Young piglets with central nervous system (CNS) lesions are often found in lateral recumbency and paddling. Older pigs have a wider variety of CNS type signs that include ataxia, opisthotonus, incoordination, tremors, convulsions, blindness and deafness. Pigs with polyarthritis have swollen joints and are lame. In some outbreaks, respiratory signs associated with pneumonia may occur. Both morbidity and mortality vary widely and are affected by treatment. *Streptococcus suis*, much like *Pasteurella multocida*, is ubiquitous in swine and a frequent secondary contributor to pneumonia.

Lesions

There often is reddening of the skin and modest enlargement of lymph nodes. Pigs that die suddenly often have fibrinopurulent meningitis microscopically, seen grossly as visible clouding of leptomeninges of the brain. In septicemic cases there may be slight enlargement of the spleen and petechial hemorrhages on the kidneys or other organs. With polyarthritis there is enlargement of joints that contain turbid synovial fluid. *Streptococcus suis* pneumonia, often secondary, has a bronchogenic distribution pattern. Predominance of any one of these lesions varies in outbreaks. Polyserositis is quite common. Other lesions seen in chronic cases include endocarditis (usually on the mitral valve), myocarditis and fibrinopurulent to fibrous pericarditis.

Diagnosis

A tentative diagnosis often can be made on the basis of history, signs, lesions and the demonstration of Gram-positive cocci in the lesions. Confirmation should be made through culture and identification of the streptococci. Both pathogenic and nonpathogenic strains can be recovered from pigs on most farms so presence of the organism, especially in an unexpected area, in addition to presentation of a typical clinical picture is important in establishing the correct diagnosis. If convenient, the capsular type should be determined since that can assist in selecting an appropriate vaccine. The predominate capsular type may change over time within a farm so periodic typing of *S. suis* organisms recovered from affected pigs may have value as an epidemiologic tool. Outbreaks are frequently associated with a variety of infectious and non-infectious risk factors so a complete diagnostic evaluation of agents and the environment is usually warranted.

Control

At present there are no highly effective measures for control of *S. suis*. Elimination of stresses, particularly overcrowding, poor ventilation, high humidity, and inadequate sanitation should be part of the strategy. The all in/all out system with emphasis on age segregation, multiple site rearing and strict sanitation of facilities and instruments used in processing piglets may be beneficial. Control of primary diseases (PRRS, influenza, pseudorabies, mycoplasmosis, etc.) that interact with *S. suis* is important. It may reduce incidence and improve response to treatment.

Affected pigs should be treated individually and as early as possible with injectable antibiotics. Systemically absorbed antibiotics are sometimes pulsed for a few days in feed or water to groups experiencing high morbidity. Some strains of *S. suis* are resistant to many antibiotics (particularly tetracyclines) so sensitivity tests are helpful in selecting a therapeutic agent. Because the type of *S. suis* may differ in consecutive outbreaks, sensitivity tests often need to be repeated.

Both commercial antisera and vaccines are available and are of value. The capsular type of the product used should be the same as the type causing the disease. Not all vaccines have been effective, perhaps because the product used was not appropriate for the serotype causing the problem or because of shift to another predominant serotype within the herd. Vaccination of sows prior to farrowing may be more effective and less costly than vaccinating the pigs for control in suckling piglets but is of less value for control of postweaning streptococcosis.

Streptococcus suis can be an important zoonotic pathogen with spread generally thought to be a result of direct inoculation through skin wounds. A large outbreak of Type 2 infection in humans was reported from China in 2005 that included a case fatality rate of approximately 18%.

Swine Dysentery and Spirochaetal Colitis

(*Brachyspira* [previously *Serpulina* and *Treponema*] *hyodysenteriae* and *Brachyspira pilosicoli*)

Definition

Swine dysentery (SD) is a severe, infectious disease characterized by mucohemorrhagic diarrhea and marked inflammation limited to the large intestine (cecum and/or colon). Spirochaetal colitis (SC) causes milder colitis in young pigs.

Occurrence

Swine dysentery (SD) occurs only in swine although the etiologic agent infects and persists in rodents. All ages of swine may have SD although it seldom is apparent in piglets less than three weeks old. The disease occurs more frequently during the growing/finishing periods. Swine dysentery occurs worldwide in the major swine-raising countries and can cause very significant economic losses on affected herds. In the United States, SD now occurs only occasionally because of successful eradication and/or effective manure removal techniques. Outbreaks occur throughout the year, more often in late summer and early fall. With the increased interest in niche pork production (e.g. organic, antibiotic free) in the US, there has been an increase in incidence of SD in these systems.

Spirochaetal colitis associated with *Brachyspira pilosicoli* also has worldwide distribution, causing a milder, non-hemorrhagic colitis.

Historical information

Swine dysentery was first reported in 1921. Subsequently it was reported from many swine-raising countries throughout the world. The etiology remained unknown until 1971. Much of the extensive research on the disease was reported during the 1970s and 1980s. Spirochaetal colitis associated with *Brachyspira pilosicoli* was described subsequent to SD.

Prior to the discovery of organic arsenicals as an effective treatment and preventative, SD caused disastrous losses among swine herds. Improved methods of control have markedly reduced losses in the US, although SD is still an important disease in some parts of the world. Methods of elimination of SD from swine herds have been well described and the establishment of a national eradication program has been considered, but lack of a sensitive monitoring test remains a problem.

Etiology

Brachyspira (previously, *Serpulina* or *Treponema*) *hyodysenteriae*, a spirochete, is the etiologic agent. It has axial filaments, is Gram-negative, anaerobic and the most pathogenic strains are strongly beta-hemolytic. There are a few avirulent or weakly beta-hemolytic *Brachyspira* strains that are predominantly nonpathogenic. Other organisms in the large intestine, especially anaerobes, may facilitate colonization and lesion formation. *Brachyspira hyodysenteriae* has the ability to survive under a wide range of environmental conditions but is susceptible to heat, ultraviolet (UV) light, and desiccation, as well as soaps and disinfectants. Other spirochetes, especially *B. innocens* and *B. pilosicoli* are found in the large intestine of many swine and are easily mistaken for *B. hyodysenteriae.*

While considering a diagnosis of swine dysentery, one should be aware of recent work in describing a nonfatal, non-bloody, diarrheal disease in swine caused by *Brachyspira* (*Serpulina*) *pilosicoli.* This agent appears to be common in swine populations and is an occasional cause of catarrhal colitis in young growing swine. Virtually all statements related to *B. hyodysenteriae* are also true for *B. pilosicoli* with the exception that disease caused by the latter is much milder.

Epidemiology

Transmission of *B. hyodysenteriae* is by ingestion of infectious feces. It can persist in lagoon water for at least two months, moist feces for two months, and soil for 18 days. Mice have been reported to shed *B. hyodysenteriae* for 180 days and dogs for 13 days. The organism can be transmitted by birds, flies, and fomites. Carrier swine can transmit the agent for at least 90 days. Clinically normal, purchased carriers, including breeding stock, often are the source of initial exposure. Carrier sows often transmit to their piglets. Infected mice on premises may also be a source of infection.

Pathogenesis

Brachyspira hyodysenteriae is ingested with clinical signs developing 5-21 days later; incubation period is dependent upon dose but the infective dose is quite small. The organism reaches the large intestine where it colonizes, proliferates, penetrates the mucus layer and becomes closely associated with epithelial cells. Invasion may not be essential for lesion production. The exact mechanism of tissue destruction is not known but lipopolysaccharide in the organism probably is involved. Also, *B. hyodysenteriae* produces two known toxins and a hemolysin that may play roles. In typical lesions the organisms can be seen within epithelial cells and occasionally in the lamina propria. Lack of lesions at other sites suggests the entire pathogenesis is associated with the cecal and colonic lesions. B. pilosicoli appears to exert pathogenic effect by attachment to enterocytes and microerosion of epithelium.

Systemic effects presumably are the result of fluid and electrolyte imbalance caused by colitis. Fluid imbalance is the result of failure of the colon to absorb fluid, much of it from endogenous secretions, and explains the progressive dehydration and deaths that occur. Peracute deaths occasionally occur, perhaps caused by the toxins.

Clinical signs

Diarrhea, usually with gray to yellow, mucoid feces often is the first sign noticed. With SD, diarrhea continues and quickly becomes mucohemorrhagic, with excess mucus and fresh blood apparent. In a small percent of the pigs, diarrhea may be preceded by tail twitching or a humped, gaunt appearance. Fresh, red blood in mucus-containing feces often is profuse and the perineal area may become blood stained. Signs that follow prolonged diarrhea are those associated with dehydration. These include sunken eyes, marked weakness, hollow flanks and weight loss. In advanced cases, appetite is erratic but the animals continue to drink. Advanced cases remain unthrifty, even with treatment. Occasionally, sudden death is observed. In untreated herds morbidity is high and mortality can approach 50%.

Spirochaetal colitis is generally seen as a mild persistent diarrhea with mucus. Affected pigs may be less thrifty but effects on growth performance may not be overtly obvious.

Lesions

Lesions are limited to large intestine, except for dehydration and the nonspecific reddening of the gastric mucosa. The mesentery and serosa are edematous and the serosa is rather opaque. Any or all parts of the large intestine (cecum, spiral colon, rectum) may be affected. It is heavy, thick walled, congested and edematous. The mucosa is thrown into folds and is covered, diffusely or in patches, with a layer of fibrin, necrotic debris and mucus. There often are flecks of blood in the mucus or on uncovered mucosa. The colon contains fibrinonecrotic debris and excessive mucus, often mixed with blood.

In acute cases the mucosa of the affected large intestine is reddened, edematous and swollen. There may be only small amounts of fibrin but excessive mucus. Blood usually can be seen in the feces. Pigs that die suddenly may be in surprisingly thrifty condition although lesions in the large intestine are extensive.

Microscopically, there is moderate nonsuppurative colitis and typhlitis, mucosal metaplasia, edema, and superficial epithelial necrosis. Spiral-shaped organisms can be demonstrated within crypts, enterocytes, and debris by silver stain.

Lesions of spirochaetal colitis are milder, with mild hyperemia and excess mucus observed on the mucosa of large intestine. Microscopically, there may be abundant spiral-shaped organisms colonizing epithelium, accompanied by mild nonsuppurative inflammation.

Diagnosis

A field diagnosis of SD often can be made on the basis of clinical signs and typical gross lesions. A simple aid in diagnosis is the demonstration of many spirochetes in stained smears made from colonic scrapings. *Brachyspira hyodysenteriae* is weakly Gram-negative so organisms are best demonstrated with crystal violet or Victoria blue 4-R stains. Other spirochetes are easily mistaken for *B. hyodysenteriae*, so it is advisable to get laboratory confirmation of the diagnosis, especially if the outbreak is an initial one or there is doubt about the diagnosis. *B. hyodysenteriae* often can be cultured and identified from rectal swabs or colonic scrapings from acutely affected, unmedicated pigs. Biochemical differentiation of pathogenic and nonpathogenic strains can be challenging. Polymerase chain reaction (PCR) techniques are available for detection of the organism and provide differentiation to the species level; their use is encouraged.

Several diarrheal diseases of swine must be differentiated from SD. These include proliferative enteritis, whipworm infestation, gastric ulcers, spirochaetal colitis (*B. pilosicoli*), and salmonellosis. Severe whipworm infections mimic mucohemorrhagic SD and worms are not grossly visible until three to four weeks after infestation. Salmonellosis lesions usually are not confined to the large intestine, as are swine dysentery lesions. Lesions of salmonellosis tend to extend deeper into the mucosa as ulcers and may be patchy in distribution with less mucus. Necropsy of several pigs and microscopic study of the colon often are helpful in separating the two diseases. Dual infections can occur. Spirochaetal colitis is best diagnosed by necropsy of acutely affected pigs, histopathology, isolation of the weakly beta-hemolytic causative organism, and definitive identification biochemically or by PCR.

Control

Preventing the introduction of *B. hyodysenteriae* to negative herds is a high priority. Additions to the herd should be only from herds known to be free of swine dysentery. They should be added only after a quarantine period of 30-60 days. Some veterinarians recommend treating high-risk animals with tiamulin or carbadox during quarantine to reduce the possibility of carriers being introduced.

Three methods are used to eliminate swine dysentery and have been quite successful in the US. Early weaned piglets (< three weeks) taken to a clean site and raised there usually remain free of *B. hyodysenteriae*. Meanwhile, the infected herd can be marketed, and the facilities cleaned and disinfected. This method allows one to retain valuable genetic stock. Segregated rearing with all in/all out production techniques has been quite successful in eliminating SD.

A second method relies on medication. Reduction of a herd to a minimal number of animals, followed by intensive treatment of those retained, is often used. Debilitated animals must be disposed of since they may not consume enough medicated feed or water. Prolonged, intensive treatment is expensive so numbers of swine to be treated should be minimized. Three widely used therapeutic agents include carbadox, lincomycin and tiamulin. Directions for their use should be followed carefully and every animal must be treated.

The third method of complete depopulation may be useful on premises with endemic swine dysentery where biosecurity and sanitation are difficult to implement. Depopulation should be done during warm, dry weather. During depopulation all facilities and equipment should be thoroughly cleaned and disinfected. The premises should be left vacant for at least two weeks, depending on the weather and level of achievable sanitation. *Brachyspira hyodysenteriae* usually will not survive for more than two weeks in soil or grass pens kept dry and relatively free of feces during dry, warm weather. Repopulation should be made with swine free of SD.

Any effort to eradicate SD requires an initial accurate diagnosis of SD, a commitment from the owners, and initial agreement on a protocol for accomplishing eradication and ongoing veterinary supervision. The eradication effort should be made during the warmest time of the year. A professionally-managed rodent control program is essential. Eradication must be coordinated with pig flow so that thorough cleaning and disinfection can be accomplished when the premises are vacant or the population minimal. If infected animals must be retained during the effort, a barrier system must be set up to separate clean from potentially contaminated areas.

Producers trying to control, but not eliminate infection with endemic swine dysentery can use preventive and therapeutic levels of antibiotics administered in feed and/or water. Those herds often can be treated intermittently to advantage. Although several products are FDA-approved for swine dysentery, carbadox, lincomycin, and tiamulin seem to be most effective. Antibiotic resistance is an increasing problem with this organism, making control programs (as opposed to elimination) a poor long term strategy. Vaccination has not proved to be reliably effective in control or elimination programs.

Control of *B. pilosicoli* should follow the same principals of sanitation and husbandry. The disease usually responds favorably to the antimicrobials listed for swine dysentery.

Tuberculosis

Definition

This is a chronic, granulomatous disease of swine, poultry, wild birds, many domestic and wild animals and people.

Occurrence

Tuberculosis (TB) occurs frequently in man, domestic and wild animals, poultry and wild birds. It occurs in almost all vertebrates and in some cold-blooded animals. In the US, the disease in domestic species and people occurs less often than in developing countries. The disease is present worldwide throughout the year.

In 1995, the incidence of TB condemnations in 100 million swine slaughtered in federally inspected abattoirs of the US was 0.003%.

Historical information

In the United States, TB once was a common disease of farm poultry flocks, cattle, swine and people. Swine often were exposed to other infected species or materials contaminated by them.

A major effort to eradicate tuberculosis in cattle and in people markedly reduced incidence of the types of tuberculosis usually seen in cattle and people. Changes in poultry production largely eliminated the raising of farm poultry flocks, which was the usual source of exposure of swine. A traceback system identified the source of infected swine for slaughter and reduced infection at points of origin. As a consequence of these measures, TB in swine was reduced substantially in incidence. Reduction was achieved without an eradication program directed specifically at swine or poultry.

Increasing prevalence of TB in immunocompromised people, coupled with resistance of tuberculosis to many therapeutic agents, is now of great public health concern. Avian type TB once was believed to be rare in people but more recently some of the serovars of avian type TB found in confinement-raised swine have been found in people. At slaughter, those serovars have caused marked condemnation losses to pork producers. These developments may translate into increased concern for TB in both swine and poultry.

Etiology

Classification of the tuberculosis bacteria (mycobacteria) is incomplete; a numerical system of classification is emerging but classical terminology is used here.

As a genus, mycobacteria are Gram-positive, acid fast bacilli. They are highly resistant to most environmental factors, many disinfectants and a large and increasing number of antibiotics. Avian type mycobacteria (*Mycobacterium avium*) have survived for more than four years in poultry lot soil, in cages, and in sawdust used as litter.

The three *Mycobacterium* species that cause tuberculosis in swine are *Mycobacterium avium*, *Mycobacterium bovis* and *Mycobacterium tuberculosis*. These three species infect poultry, cattle and people, respectively. However, each of these three occasionally infects other animal species.

Mycobacterium avium usually is the organism that infects swine. There are 19 known serovars. In the US serovars l, 2, 4 and 8 are the most common isolates from swine. Serovars 4 and 8 have been found in poultry, large confined swine herds and people.

Epidemiology

The marked resistance of mycobacteria to environmental factors makes contaminated premises a long-term threat to swine. The TB organisms usually are spread to swine by tuberculosis-infected poultry, wild birds, cattle or people, or by soil or bedding materials contaminated by them. The route of exposure usually is by ingestion although spread by inhalation occurs occasionally. Infectious feeds that have spread TB bacilli to swine include offal from infected poultry and cattle, uncooked garbage, unpasteurized milk and dairy products. Exposure of swine to lots contaminated by the feces of tuberculosis-infected poultry often has led to their infection by *M. avium*.

Other less common but proven routes of exposure include exposure to serovars of avian type contained in sawdust or wood shavings used as bedding, congenital exposure of fetuses of infected, pregnant sows, and animal-to-animal exposure among swine. Some infected swine have TB lesions in their tonsils or intestine and shed the organisms in their feces.

Pathogenesis

The complex lipid nature of the organisms may explain the difficulties that body defenses have in destroying mycobacteria though phagocytosis and oxidative killing. In mononuclear phagocytes, toxic lipids in the mycobacteria, or factors released by them, appear to interfere with phagolysosome formation or to inactivate lysosomal enzymes. If macrophages fail to destroy ingested mycobacteria, they can carry them to other sites. There, the bacteria are liberated upon death of the macrophages and released organisms set up new foci of infection.

In swine, TB bacilli appear to infect the tonsils and intestinal mucosa initially and then spread to the regional lymph nodes, especially those of the cervical area, less often to mesenteric nodes. Lesions in the nodes tend to develop slowly and, in most cases, the bacilli are successfully walled off. Only occasionally does the infection generalize, usually in older breeding stock infected with *M. bovis*.

Clinical signs

In swine with localized TB infections, there usually are no signs. Since most swine are slaughtered at an early age, there is little time for generalization of infection and the appearance of signs. Condemnation of carcasses at slaughter is the usual presentation. In older breeding stock, TB generalization does occur occasionally. Affected animals tend to waste away despite adequate feed. They eventually become emaciated and may die from tuberculosis.

Lesions

In localized TB, grossly visible lesions usually are apparent only in cervical, submaxillary or mesenteric lymph nodes. Lesions vary considerably in appearance, depending on the type of infection. Localized avian and human type infections tend to produce enlarged, firm nodes with no discrete purulent foci. Calcification is seldom apparent and lesions are not easily enucleated. Nodes affected by *M. bovis* tend to be well encapsulated, relatively easy to enucleate, and there often is marked calcification in the lesions.

Mycobacterium bovis tends to generalize more readily than do other forms of tuberculosis. Lesions in the organs vary considerably. Initially, the lesions are miliary and widely distributed. Those in the lungs tend to develop along pleural and septal lymphatics and resemble dewdrops. Those in the liver tend to have caseated or liquefied centers. Splenic lesions occur commonly and, when well developed, they often protrude. Serous membranes seldom are affected.

It is not possible to accurately identify tuberculosis, or the particular variety of tuberculosis on the basis of gross or microscopic lesions. Lesions, including discrete granulomas containing acid-fast organisms, can be caused by other agents and are easily mistaken as tuberculosis.

Diagnosis

A presumptive diagnosis often can be made on the basis of history, study of gross and microscopic lesions and the presence of acid-fast bacteria within discrete granulomas or granulomatous tissue. However, errors will be made. Firm, unequivocal diagnosis can be made only after isolation, identification and typing of the bacteria. Polymerase chain reaction (PCR) and immunohistochemistry (IHC) are increasingly useful for confirmation.

Control

Prevention is by avoiding exposure of swine to TB bacilli (see under Epidemiology). Eradication of avian TB would reduce the likelihood of exposure to TB bacilli but is not possible. Raising either swine or poultry in confinement can reduce the most common exposure of swine to infection. Conversely, close confinement of swine with careless exposure to wild birds or poultry can provide an opportunity for greater exposure. All swine, as well as bedding, should be protected from birds.

No effort should be made to treat TB in swine.

Section II

Domestic Viral Diseases

Encephalomyocarditis

Definition
Encephalomyocarditis (EMC) is a disease caused by a viral infection. Infection with EMC viruses is common in susceptible species, but clinical disease is unusual in domestic animals and humans.

Occurrence
Susceptible species include humans, primates, many species of rodents, marsupials, mongoose species, and several species of birds. In zoos, rapidly fatal infections have been reported in elephants, primates, and artiodactyls. Horses, cattle, swine, dogs, and cats are susceptible to infection, but except for swine, there is no clear evidence that EMC viruses are significant pathogens of domesticated species.

The encephalomyocarditis group of viruses (EMCV) is present throughout the world. Infection is common but clinical disease is rare in domestic animals and humans. A survey of 104 swine herds in Iowa found 13.8% of breeding stock and 8.5% of finishers had serum-neutralizing antibodies against EMCV. Approximately 90% of herds had one or more animals with antibody titers. Other serosurveys have reported similar, or higher, prevalence rates in swine.

Historical information
Columbia SK virus, the first strain of EMCV identified, was described in 1940. It was initially postulated to be a previously unrecognized strain of poliovirus, but this was later shown not to be the case. Infection in swine was not reported until outbreaks occurred in Panama (1958) and Florida (1960). Subsequently, clinical EMC was reported in Australia, Brazil, Cuba, Greece, New Zealand, and North America.

Considerable research on the EMC viruses in swine was conducted up to the mid 1990s. Much of the interest in EMC was generated because of an erroneous association with "mystery swine disease," later proven to be caused by porcine reproductive and respiratory syndrome virus (PRRSV). Porcine reproductive and respiratory syndrome virus may have caused some outbreaks previously attributed to EMC. At present, the significance of EMC as a swine pathogen in the US is dubious.

Etiology
The EMC group of viruses is classified in the genus Cardiovirus in the Picornaviridae family. They are nonenveloped, single-stranded RNA viruses and strains vary in virulence. These hemagglutinating viruses are stable and can be grown in cell cultures derived from several animal species. Areas contaminated with the EMC viruses can be disinfected with iodine-based disinfectants or 0.5 ppm residual chlorine.

Epidemiology
Rats and mice are commonly considered to be the principal reservoirs of the virus, although the experimental evidence does not support this hypothesis. Transmission of EMC virus among rodent species is difficult to achieve and a chronic intestinal carrier state, a keystone epidemiologic feature in closely related picornaviruses (i.e. polioviruses or enteroviruses), does not occur. Infected rodents excrete virus and their diseased carcasses contain large amounts of virus. Presumably, swine are infected by ingesting feed or water contaminated by rats, mice, or the carcasses of animals that died from EMC. Infected swine excrete virus for about 9 days but it is not clear that they play an important role in transmission to other pigs. Virus has been isolated from certain tick and mosquito species, but vector competency studies have not shown transmission from infected arthropods.

Pathogenesis
Following experimental oral infection of piglets, viremia occurs. Lymphoid tissues contain virus and probably are the major sites of virus replication. The highest titers of virus occur in damaged heart muscle. Most deaths probably are related to right heart failure. Transplacental infections occur in fetuses near full term and many develop myocardial lesions. Pigs that survive develop antibodies that persist for long periods.

Clinical signs
Infection in swine is usually subclinical, but in rare cases it produces myocarditis and high mortality in nursing pigs and/or reproductive failure in dams. For unknown reasons, clinical outbreaks in swine generally occur in tropical or semi-tropical climates. Clinical disease in young piglets is often characterized by an acute course and sudden death. Less acute cases have respiratory signs with dyspnea, fever, anorexia, depression, trembling, staggering and paralysis. Mortality may approach 100% in neonatal and nursing pigs. Older pigs and adults usually have subclinical infection but some mortality may occur, even among adults. In pregnant sows and gilts, there are mid-to-near term abortions with an increase in stillbirths and mummified fetuses.

Lesions
The characteristic gross lesions seen in acute disease are discrete, white, focal discolorations of the myocardium, at times accompanied by a nonsuppurative meningoencephalitis. The lesions in young piglets are those of right heart failure, including hepatomegaly, hydropericardium, hydrothorax, pulmonary edema and ascites. The heart may be enlarged, flabby, and pale red with subepicardial, petechial hemorrhages. Lesions are most marked in the right ventricle where there may be discrete yellow or white foci or diffuse, pale areas of myocardial necrosis. Similar myocardial lesions may be visible in the heart of late-aborted fetuses. Microscopic lesions include focal nonsuppurative interstitial myocarditis and myocardial necrosis; infiltration of small numbers of neutrophils may be evident.

Diagnosis

Disease associated with EMC is rare but should be considered in cases where there is marked dyspnea and sudden deaths in preweaning age piglets, high preweaning mortality and an increase in late term abortions, or gross and/or microscopic myocardial lesions. Myocardial lesions must be differentiated from those of PRRSV, mulberry heart disease, toxoplasmosis, bacterial septicemia, and cardiac infarcts.

Definitive diagnosis requires isolation and identification of the virus, coupled with observation of typical lesions. The virus usually is isolated from the myocardium or spleen of acute cases in young piglets. A number of serologic assays (serum neutralization [SN], hemagglutination inhibition [HI], agar gel immunodiffusion [AGID], enzyme-linked immunosorbent assay [ELISA], latex agglutination) have been developed for the antibody detection. The SN assay is widely available and has been shown to be specific for antibodies against EMCV. No cross-neutralizing activity was found between EMCV and 62 human enterovirus serotypes or 11 porcine enterovirus serotypes. Serum neutralizing antibodies may persist for an extended period of time, so serologic evidence of recent infection requires demonstrating a 4-fold increase in neutralizing antibody titers in convalescent versus acute sera. Molecular diagnostic techniques (nucleic acid probe, polymerase chain reaction [PCR]) have been described, but are not widely available.

Control

Until EMC is definitely demonstrated to be a significant cause of disease, it is better ignored. Elimination or reduction of feral rodent populations is recommended in order to minimize environmental contamination with virus. Feeds from all sources should be properly stored and kept free of contamination by rodents. Pigs from premises known to have EMC should not be added to known negative herds. Pigs, rodents, and other animals that have died should be removed promptly to avoid transmission through ingestion. Basic hygienic and sanitary practices should be followed. An inactivated vaccine is commercially available but its use should be clearly justified. There is no specific treatment.

Hemagglutinating Encephalomyelitis
(Vomiting and Wasting Disease)

Definition
A disease seen in pigs less than four weeks old, characterized by signs that include vomiting, wasting and, perhaps, neurologic signs.

Occurrence
Hemagglutinating encephalomyelitis (HE) occurs only in swine. The disease occurs in most major swine-raising countries but tends to be quite sporadic. Infection is clinically silent except in piglets less than four weeks old. In these, the disease occurs as an acute outbreak affecting most piglets in litters of nonimmune dams.

Historical information
In 1959 an encephalomyelitis of suckling pigs was reported in Ontario, Canada. In 1962, other investigators reported a hemagglutinating virus producing encephalomyelitis in baby pigs. In 1969, vomiting and wasting disease, similar in many respects to the encephalomyelitis reported in Canada, was reported in England. Viruses from the outbreaks later were proven to be similar or identical.

Much of the research on HE infection in swine was completed in the 1970s and 1980s. Epidemiologic studies have shown the virus to be widespread in the US. However, clinical outbreaks seldom occur and the disease is of modest economic importance.

Etiology
Two overlapping syndromes are caused by a single hemagglutinating coronavirus. The virus can be grown in several porcine cell culture systems and hemagglutinates erythrocytes from several kinds of animals. Only one serotype of the virus is recognized. Differences in strain virulence, along with differences in susceptibility, are responsible for the two syndromes. The virus is moderately resistant to destructive environmental factors.

Epidemiology
Only pigs are susceptible. Transmission of virus is presumably through actively infected or carrier swine. Exposure is probably through infectious nasal secretions or aerosol. Most large breeding herds in major swine-raising countries are endemically infected. In most swine herds, immune sows provide colostral antibody that protects their piglets for 4-18 weeks. Passive immunity in the growing pigs is replaced by active immunity as a consequence of exposure to virus in the environment followed by subclinical infection. Clinically apparent disease develops only when young piglets from nonimmune sows are exposed.

Pathogenesis
Transmitted virus replicates in the nasal epithelial mucosa, tonsils, lungs and small intestine and spreads via the peripheral nervous system to the central nervous system (CNS). Viremia is probably of little significance in spread. In the CNS, virus localizes first in nuclei in the medulla oblongata but later progresses to the brain stem, spinal cord and sometimes to the cerebrum and cerebellum. The virus produces lesions in a variety of nuclei, ganglia and plexi (trigeminal ganglion, vagal sensory nuclei, some brain stem nuclei, intramural plexi of the stomach). Clinical signs vary, depending upon which nuclei are affected by the virus. Death occurs whenever a vital nucleus ceases to function.

Clinical signs
Vomiting and wasting syndrome: Sneezing and coughing may occur at onset. Within a few days, vomiting of milk and retching are prominent signs. The young pigs dehydrate rapidly and often grind their teeth. When water is supplied, piglets mouth it but drink little, presumably because of pharyngeal paralysis. After a few days they exhibit dyspnea, cyanosis, coma and die.

Pigs in older litters survive longer but continue to vomit occasionally. The anterior abdomen of some of them may become distended, presumably from impaired emptying and accumulation of gas. Most affected piglets waste away over a few weeks and die. The few that survive remain unthrifty. Morbidity and mortality in both syndromes approaches 100% in affected litters.

Encephalomyelitis syndrome: Initial signs are similar to those in the above syndrome. Vomiting and retching occur less often and lead to less dehydration. In one to three days, any of a variety of signs of encephalomyelitis appear. These may include: stilted gait, muscle tremors, nystagmus, blindness, opisthotonus, convulsions, and progressive paresis leading to recumbency with paddling of the legs. Occasional pigs walk backwards and assume a dog-sitting position. Affected pigs soon weaken, pass into coma and die. In some litters of older pigs, there may be only transient posterior paresis followed by recovery.

Lesions
Lesions are similar in the two syndromes. Chronically infected pigs have cachexia and there may be distension of the anterior abdomen by excessive gas in the stomach.

Microscopic lesions include a nonsuppurative encephalitis affecting the gray matter of the medulla and brain stem. The frequency of lesions at specific sites may vary in the two syndromes. There is inflammation of the trigeminal, paravertebral and autonomic ganglia. Also, ganglia in the stomach wall, mostly in the pyloric area, may show degeneration.

Diagnosis
The history, signs, and age group affected may suggest the diagnosis. Microscopic lesions, also, are helpful in diagnosis. However,

for definitive diagnosis the virus should be isolated and identified. Isolation can best be made from the brain stem of piglets showing signs for less than two days. Paired early and late serum samples sometimes can be used to show a rise in antibody titer against the infection. The first blood samples should be taken early in the course of the disease since antibody levels rise quickly. There does not appear to be serologic cross-reaction with other porcine coronaviruses (transmissible gastroenteritis [TGE], porcine respiratory coronavirus [PRCV]).

Control

Hyperimmune serum or serum from swine of an immune herd can be given for prevention during the early stages of an outbreak. However, outbreaks run their course so rapidly (two to three weeks), the time necessary for diagnosis and obtaining serum makes this impractical.

Once the virus is introduced, it persists in the herd. Most breeding stock has been exposed, has developed an active immunity and provides adequate passive immunity for their piglets.

There is no effective treatment.

Inclusion Body Rhinitis
(Porcine Cytomegalovirus Infection)

Definition
A viral infection usually manifested in nursing or newly-weaned piglets as a rhinitis and conjunctivitis accompanied by sneezing and nasal discharge. Infection of pregnant, naïve sows may lead to delivery of dead, mummified, stillborn or weak piglets.

Occurrence
Porcine cytomegalovirus (PCMV), also known as inclusion body rhinitis (IBR) occurs in all age groups of previously uninfected swine, including developing fetuses. PCMV occurs only in pigs although similar infections with related viruses occur in many other species, including people. PCMV occurs worldwide in the major swine-raising countries. Infection is common but often is inapparent when herd immunity is present or in pigs over six weeks old.

Historical information
A rhinitis of pigs accompanied by inclusion bodies was described in 1955. In 1961 the disease was identified as a transplacental infection of fetal pigs. Beginning in the early 1960s and extending into the late 1980s, research reports provided details on the disease and its manifestations in all ages of swine as well as characteristics of the virus that causes the disease. There has been interest in a possible relationship of PCMV to reproductive failure in dams and early neonatal losses. It has been suspected of predisposing swine to other respiratory diseases, especially atrophic rhinitis. Losses from PCMV are small. The disease and infection are largely ignored by swine raisers.

Etiology
Porcine cytomegalovirus causes inclusion body rhinitis. The cytomegaloviruses are a subgroup of the herpesviruses. They have many of the characteristics of herpesviruses, including the ability to induce latent infection in carriers that can later be reactivated by stress. PCMV can be propagated in cell culture. In several epithelial type cells of swine the virus causes marked cell enlargement and formation of large intranuclear inclusion bodies.

Epidemiology
Serologic testing has shown that many herds are serologically positive to PCMV. The presence of the virus within a herd often is unrecognized because many sows are immune, show no signs of infection, and colostral antibodies protect their young piglets from lesions as they are infected.

Virus is shed during and for some time after infection. Many infected piglets three to eight weeks old shed virus. Virus is shed in nasal and ocular secretions, urine and the aerosol created by sneezing and coughing. Transmission of virus is, presumably, through inhalation or ingestion of virus. Many recovered animals have virus sequestered as a latent infection and can then become shedders if severely stressed. These carriers then disseminate virus while mixed with susceptible swine.

Experimentally, and probably naturally, the virus sometimes crosses the placenta to infect developing fetuses. Infected fetuses may be killed, mummified, stillborn or born alive as infected, weak piglets. Infected piglets then spread virus to susceptible piglets.

Pathogenesis
The primary site of virus replication is believed to be in the nasal mucous glands or the lachrymal or Harderian glands. Destruction of their cells results in a marked rhinitis and conjunctivitis.

Viremia follows replication. The virus localizes in epithelial and endothelial cells at many sites as well as within macrophages and reticuloendothelial cells. The intracellular virus causes marked enlargement and destruction of many infected cells but persists and is tolerated by other cells. Regeneration can occur in some simple glands by proliferation and differentiation of ductal cells. Endothelial cell damage and necrosis is believed to be responsible for the petechial hemorrhages and edema that accompany IBR. Bone marrow damage is suspected of causing anemia in neonates. Widespread damage caused by the virus or secondary infections can lead to death.

Clinical signs
The disease usually is observed in one to five week old pigs. In suckling pigs, especially pigs less than three weeks old, signs include mucopurulent rhinitis accompanied by violent sneezing, respiratory distress, conjunctivitis, shivering, perhaps mouth breathing, and a variable death loss. Although unusual, mortality can be high in pigs born to naïve gilts or sows, or if PCMV is complicated by other diseases.

Infected neonatal piglets appear weak, anemic or stunted and there may be edema around the throat and tarsal joints. Signs in older pigs or dams with viremia may include listlessness and mild anorexia or may be inapparent.

Fetal mummification, stillbirths, neonatal deaths and failure of piglets to thrive have been associated with infection of naïve, pregnant sows. Evidence that IBR caused these has been accumulated through field observations and is supported by related research.

Lesions
In nursing piglets, the most commonly recognized gross lesion is mucopurulent exudate in, and perhaps obstructing, nasal passages. Complications sometimes include sinusitis, otitis media or pneumonia. In neonatal pigs, petechial hemorrhages and subcutaneous edema can occur. Effusions in the thorax, abdomen and pericardial

sac and edema of the lungs often are present. Microscopically, intranuclear inclusions usually can be found in nasal mucous glands, Harderian glands and lachrymal glands of nursing pigs. They may be present in renal glomeruli and tubular epithelium, liver, capillary endothelium, choroid plexus, glial cells and in various epithelial type cells. Focal gliosis is common throughout the central nervous system (CNS). Inclusions sometimes can be found at several sites in fetuses.

Diagnosis

The disease usually is diagnosed after finding microscopic, basophilic intranuclear inclusions in tissues of a typical, infected piglet. Where available, an enzyme linked immunosorbent assay (ELISA) or an indirect immunofluorescent (IF) test on serum samples can be used to confirm the presence of PCMV in a herd. If reproductive problems have occurred in a herd, PCMV will need to be differentiated from other reproductive diseases, especially parvoviral infection, pseudorabies (PRV) and porcine reproductive and respiratory syndrome (PRRS).

Control

Because the disease seldom is recognized as a cause of severe loss, control measures often are ignored. Growing pigs usually are protected from large losses by antibodies provided by their immune dams. As piglets grow, they are exposed to virus in the environment and respond by producing their own antibodies.

Environmental conditions, if poor, should be improved. Herd immunity via acclimatization of breeding stock is commonly practiced. There is no known effective treatment or medication. Antibiotics may be useful to control concurrent diseases or secondary bacterial infections.

Influenza (Swine Influenza; Swine Flu)

Definition

Swine influenza is a rapidly spreading viral disease characterized by sudden onset of fever, occulonasal discharge, prostration and weakness, followed by paroxysmal coughing over a relatively short course of 5-7 days, and relatively low mortality in uncomplicated outbreaks.

Occurrence

In the United States, swine influenza (SIV) is common and widespread. Serologic surveys show that nearly all of the herds in the Midwest have antibodies to SIV.

Swine influenza occurs in swine of all ages. Outbreaks once were seen mainly in the fall and winter in finishing animals but now occur throughout the year and can be seen in younger, nursery age pigs. The disease is present in most major swine-raising countries.

Historical information

Swine influenza subtype H1N1 first appeared in western Illinois in 1918 during an influenza pandemic that killed an estimated 20 million people worldwide.

Increased interest in zoonoses and public health has included an intense interest in all influenza viruses. There now is clear evidence of interspecies transmission of influenza viruses among swine, chickens, ducks, turkeys, many wild birds and people. When concurrent infection of poultry or swine with 2 or more strains of virus occurs, there is potential for reassortment of segments of genetic material with development of new strains resulting (genetic "shift").

Etiology

In the United States, SIV is caused by type A influenza viruses (family Orthomyxoviridae). Swine influenza viruses have glycoprotein "spikes" on their surface that act as major surface antigens. There are 16 hemagglutinin (H) and 9 neuraminidase (N) surface glycoproteins that are numbered to help identify virus strains. The surface antigens of influenza viruses can change because of antigenic drift, reassortment of genes during concurrent infections with different strains of virus (antigenic shift), or cross species transmission.

The classic subtype in swine, H1N1, has been the predominant subtype in swine in the US since 1918 but H3N2 and H1N2 emerged during the 1990s and have persisted as significant causes of disease in US commercial swine. These H3N2 and H1N2 isolates vary in their origin and "triple reassortment" variants that are comprised of swine, human, and avian viral genes have been identified. In Europe, subtypes H3N2, H1N1 and a second H1N1 of avian origin cause most outbreaks.

Most SIV viruses grow readily in 9-12 day old chick embryos or cell cultures and will hemagglutinate certain kinds of erythrocytes. In the laboratory this is a useful characteristic in identifying viruses through hemagglutination and hemagglutination inhibition serological tests.

Swine influenza virus probably does not survive more than two weeks outside the host and can be inactivated by many disinfectants.

Epidemiology

Acute outbreaks are a result of rapid transmission of SIV through a susceptible population, probably by nasal secretions and short-distance aerosols of infected animals; a persistent or asymptomatic carrier status does not appear to occur. Cases of human-to-pig and pig-to-human transmission have been documented to occur. The presence of antibody (maternal or active) will mitigate the severity of disease and influence the rapidity of spread through a population. Thus, swine influenza often is endemic in populations that use continuous pig flows. The importance of aerosol transmission farm-to-farm is difficult to quantify but likely occurs only over short distances.

Swine simultaneously infected with different SIV subtypes (including viruses derived from turkeys, chickens, ducks, certain waterfowl and people) may recombine to produce novel subtypes that, on rare occasion, are maintained in swine populations or transmit to other species. This "mixing vessel" effect is relatively rare and most likely to occur where there are many small farms with poultry and pigs in close association (Asia). Spread of SIV from swine to people has been documented several times but is unusual; a few deaths have been reported. Lungworms and their ova were at one time thought to be involved in the transmission of SIV but this notion has been convincingly disproven.

Pathogenesis

The SIV gains access by the nasopharyngeal route and enters respiratory epithelium where it causes inflammation with widespread degeneration and necrosis of cells lining bronchi and bronchioles. Also, virus can be demonstrated in interalveolar septa, sometimes in turbinate epithelium, and mediastinal lymph nodes. In the lung, alveolar type 2 pneumocytes are affected and produce less surfactant. This impairs phagocytosis of secondary microorganisms by alveolar macrophages. Inflammatory exudate in smaller airways sometimes blocks them, leading to atelectasis, emphysema and bronchointerstitial pneumonia. In most cases epithelial damage is repaired and the lesions resolve in five to seven days. The severity of the effect of infection is mitigated by the quantity of homologous circulating antibody (maternal or active). Most of the mortality associated with SIV is the result of secondary bacterial infections or concurrent infections with other primary agents of pneumonia.

Clinical signs

In a typical outbreak, there is a sudden onset of a marked respiratory illness affecting most pigs in the herd. Signs include prostration, weakness, fevers (104 to 106 °F), paroxysmal coughing, anorexia, and conjunctivitis with occulonasal discharge. Recovery begins about the sixth day and the herd is largely recovered in one to two weeks. Morbidity is high and mortality is low or absent in most uncomplicated outbreaks. Uncomplicated SIV usually causes little death loss but losses of weight and body condition, as well as cost of medication, can be significant. Concurrent infections with other respiratory diseases can increase mortality and culls. SIV may have a less abrupt and more prolonged clinical course when there is individual variation in immunity in the population. This endemic form of the disease course is not uncommon in the nursery and early grower period and can prove challenging to diagnose and control.

Reproductive problems occasionally associated with SIV likely are incidental to the acute illness. Infection during pregnancy may result in abortion due to acute illness in sows and sometimes small, weak litters. Transplacental infection is rare.

Lesions

The gross lesions include lobular distribution of congestion, firmness, atelectasis, emphysema and perhaps pneumonia. Gross lesions often are restricted to the apical and cardiac lobes but may affect entire lungs. Areas of atelectasis are irregular, darkened and firm. Lesions often appear as distinct, scattered lobules. Airways may contain blood-tinged exude. Regional lymph nodes are moderately enlarged. Microscopic lesions include degeneration and necrosis of portions of airway epithelium and obstruction of airways with exudate. There may be bronchointerstitial pneumonia. Marked edema and congestion of the entire lung may be present in severe cases. Necrotizing bronchiolitis is highly suggestive of SIV.

Diagnosis

A history of sudden onset of a severe respiratory illness in many animals, along with typical signs and lesions, often is adequate for a field diagnosis. It is useful to confirm the diagnosis since the disease may reappear and go unrecognized in a less typical, subacute form.

Confirmation of diagnosis can be made in several ways but detection of antigen or virus is most successful from acutely affected (febrile) pigs. The virus can be identified by fluorescent antibody technique on fresh lung sections or by immunohistochemistry techniques on formalin-fixed lung sections (successful only in acutely affected, euthanized pigs). The virus can be isolated from nasal swabs or lung tissue in chick embryos. A polymerase chain reaction (PCR) can be used to detect virus in nasal swabs or lungs. There are commercially available influenza A antigen detection kits (enzyme immunoassays) that can be used to detect SIV on nasal swabs. In some cases, paired serum samples taken early and late in an outbreak can be used to demonstrate a rising serotype-specific antibody titer to SIV. Serologic testing is complicated by the fact several subtypes of SIV can be present in a group of pigs and that most serologic tests do not sufficiently cross-react to detect antibodies of all SIV subtypes.

Because there are multiple subtypes of SIV in swine populations, mere detection of SIV is not sufficient to implement specific control strategies. The offending SIV can be subtyped by some laboratories by PCR, genetic sequencing, or serologic methods.

It is quite common to have other viral, bacterial, mycoplasmal and parasitic diseases in association with SIV, especially in outbreaks with considerable mortality.

Reproductive failure is due to the affects of acute disease in sows. The virus cannot be detected in aborted fetuses but can be detected in acutely affected sows. Serology is not a reliable method of diagnosis of reproductive failure since most sow herds will be serologically positive from previous exposure to the agent.

Control

There are no specific therapeutics for SIV. Often, antimicrobials are used to control or prevent secondary bacterial infections. Aspirin or other anti-inflammatory agents may offer relief to severely affected pigs. Treatment should emphasize providing a comfortable environment and ready access to fresh feed and water.

Prevention has depended largely on maintaining a closed herd to avoid introducing infected pigs. Inactivated vaccines are widely used in Europe and the United States. Several types of commercial vaccines are available and autogenous products are commonly used. Directions provided with the vaccine should be closely followed. Cross-protection between subtypes should not be expected in most situations.

Control of SIV in recently-weaned pigs in modern systematic production units usually requires stabilization of the breeding herd by acclimatization or vaccination. Vaccination prior to farrowing to stimulate colostral protection for the young piglets is sometimes practiced. New additions to the breeding herd should be vaccinated during their isolation period.

Successful control of SIV in the grow/finish phase of SIV-positive herds can be daunting. Nursery pigs can be vaccinated prior to moving them to the finisher. Maternal antibody interference with vaccination is a major concern in timing of vaccination since antibody levels are highly variable in populations and even low detectable antibody may interfere with immune response. There is little cross-protection between subtypes, making vaccine selection challenging. Often, the offending virus must be subtyped to aid in selection of the correct antigen.

On infected premises, the all in/all out system with cleaning and disinfection of facilities between farrowings helps prevent virus carryover as does vaccination of the breeding herd to "stabilize" the infection to prevent virus transmission to offspring. Depopulation of a continuous-flow nursery or finisher may be necessary to stop virus circulation.

Parvovirus

Definition
Porcine parvovirus (PPV) can cause reproductive failure in naïve dams. It is characterized by the occurrence of large numbers of mummified fetuses, an increase in the number of returns to estrus, small litters, failures to farrow, decreased farrowing rate, and rarely abortion.

Occurrence
Porcine parvoviral infection (PPV) is endemic in most swine herds. It usually is subclinical and a very common infection. Prior to porcine reproductive and respiratory syndrome (PRRS), PPV was probably the most commonly diagnosed infectious cause of reproductive failure in swine. Reproductive failure is much more likely to occur in gilts than in sows. PPV occurs worldwide in major swine-raising countries.

Historical information
The earliest publication about PPV occurred in 1967. Within a few years the disease was identified as a major cause of reproductive failure. Much of the research on PPV was done in the 1970s and 1980s. Most details regarding the virus and the disease it causes are now known. Losses from PPV now are well controlled, largely by vaccination, and clinical effects of PPV are now less prevalent.

Many manifestations of reproductive failure seen with PPV accompany other reproductive diseases of swine and should not be considered pathognomonic for PPV.

Etiology
The disease is caused by a porcine parvovirus (PPV). All isolates are similar antigenically. PPV is quite resistant to environmental degradation and many disinfectants. It persists for at least 4 months on contaminated premises. The virus hemagglutinates many kinds of erythrocytes, a feature useful in its laboratory identification. Porcine parvovirus does not cause diarrhea in swine although related parvoviruses do so in several other species.

Epidemiology
Parvoviral infection is endemic in most swine herds. Following infection, virus is shed in the secretions and excretions from the animal for approximately two weeks. An infected dam will disseminate virus in feces and fluids, including placental fluids and mummified fetuses. Fetuses infected during gestation can be born as infected, immunotolerant piglets that can pass the virus intermittently or continuously but the significance or likelihood of this phenomenon is unknown. Because parvovirus is quite resistant to environmental influences, contaminated facilities are an important source of exposure.

Oronasal transmission can occur among susceptible swine of all ages. Surprisingly, surveys show that many herds with endemic infection contain some animals that are susceptible.

Transplacental infection of embryos and fetuses is the result of dams failing to develop an active immunity prior to pregnancy. Passive immunity persists in some gilts beyond the time they are old enough to be bred. This interferes with their development of an active immune response to natural or vaccine exposure (active immunity usually develops following exposure of gilts to parvovirus in the environment as passive immunity wanes). Gilts with little or no immunity can be infected during their first pregnancy. If infected during pregnancy, virus may cross the placenta and infect some, or all, of their embryos or fetuses.

It is likely that PPV can be transmitted through semen or artificial insemination since it has been isolated from the semen of naturally infected boars. Also, boars may transmit virus mechanically.

Pathogenesis
Pregnant, infected dams develop a viremia during the acute phase of PPV infection. Virus then may cross some or all of the separate placentas of developing embryos or fetuses. Fetal infection during the first 35 days of gestation causes death and resorption of embryos, resulting in irregular returns to estrus or reduced litter size. Infection between 35 and 70 days of gestation results in fetal death and mummification. Since fetuses become immunologically competent by about the 70th day of gestation, fetuses older than that may successfully resist infection and survive.

After one embryo or young fetus is infected, the virus may slowly spread through the uterus and infect some or all of the others. The direct effect of PPV on the uterus, as can be seen microscopically in experimental dams, probably contributes to reproductive failure.

The death of embryos and fetuses is attributed to the direct destructive effect of parvovirus on their organs and tissues. Many kinds of cells are affected, especially mitotically active capillary endothelium and neurons. Extensive endothelial cell damage may be reflected in damage to many organs.

Clinical signs
In most swine a transient leukopenia occurs within ten days of infection with PPV. However, this and any other indication of infection are inapparent in all swine except developing fetuses. Infection of a naïve herd of pregnant females results in irregular return of bred animals to estrus, increased numbers of mummified fetuses, smaller litter size, increases in animals checked positive for pregnancy that fail to farrow, and prolonged gestation lengths. The increase in mummified fetuses after a normal gestation period is the hallmark of PPV. Abortions attributable to this virus are rare.

Lesions
Gross lesions are not apparent in the dams. The most important lesion observed with parvoviral infection is mummified fetuses. In experimentally infected dams, nonspecific microscopic and gross lesions are described but are of no diagnostic value.

Diagnosis

The lack of illness in the dams, coupled with increased mummies, irregular return to estrus and decreased litter size, primarily in gilts, is suggestive of PPV infection. A tentative diagnosis can be confirmed by demonstrating PPV antigen in the lungs of several mummified fetuses using immunofluorescent microscopy. The preferred specimen for diagnosis is the lung tissue from several mummified fetuses less than 16 cm long. Larger fetuses are not satisfactory since their tissues may contain antibody that interferes with the procedure.

It is possible but rarely practiced, to isolate the virus and identify it by hemagglutination and hemagglutination inhibition (HI) tests. Virus isolation usually is more difficult and time consuming than diagnosis through demonstration of viral antigen in fetal cells.

Sometimes antibody can be demonstrated in fluids or sera from stillborn pigs or presuckle neonatal live pigs. While this may indicate intrauterine infection with PPV, there is considerable likelihood of false positive serologic reaction from these specimens. Serology from breeding animals may be difficult to interpret since cross-sectional sampling will often reveal a wide range of titers. Demonstration of seroconversion in many gilts and sows with paired serology also may be used for a positive diagnosis but acute samples are often not available. Conversely, the absence of titers may aid in exclusion of PPV as the cause. If mummies are not available for evaluation, efforts should concentrate on gilt serology, comparing titers from unmated gilts to those exhibiting signs of infertility.

Control

Probably the best way to prevent PPV infection is to vaccinate all susceptible breeding stock twice, 2 weeks apart, several weeks before breeding. Killed vaccines are available and effective. They should stimulate an active immunity in the dams that will protect the developing fetuses. Alternatively, seronegative stock can be exposed to a herd of seropositive older stock and used for breeding only after seroconversion. Some of those should be shedding virus that would stimulate development of an active immunity. There is no effective treatment for PPV infection.

Porcine Circovirus Associated Diseases (PCVD, PCVAD)

Definition

Porcine circovirus (PCV) is a common virus of pigs found throughout the world. This DNA virus is unique for its small size (~1800 bp), circular genome, and hardiness in the environment. In the late 1990s, a novel circovirus emerged in North American swine that appeared to be genetically distinct from the prototype PCV (now referred to as PCV Type 1) and was termed PCV Type 2 (PCV2). Porcine circovirus Type 1 had been recognized for several decades as a common contaminant of laboratory cell cultures but despite being widespread in commercial swine, was nonpathogenic. The emergence of PCV2 coincided with the occurrence of a new clinical syndrome of swine referred to as postweaning multisystemic wasting syndrome (PMWS). Since its appearance, PCV2 (and PMWS) has become widely distributed in most developed swine industries around the world. The term PCVAD (porcine circovirus associated disease) is now used in North America to refer to the different disease manifestations associated with PCV2. In Europe, the acronym PCVD (porcine circovirus disease) is used instead.

Occurrence

Porcine circovirus Type 2 infection has been reported from nearly every country with a significant commercial production industry. It is strongly associated with the occurrence of PMWS and also appears to have an association with porcine dermatitis and nephropathy syndrome (PDNS), porcine respiratory disease complex (PRDC), and occasionally reproductive failure. Postweaning multisystemic wasting syndrome usually occurs in nursery or growing pigs and is diagnosed on a herd level through the occurrence of multiple features:

Microscopic	lymphocytic depletion in lymph nodes often accompanied by histiocytic infiltration
Clinical	loss of body condition in affected individuals, enlarged lymph nodes
Epidemiologic	increased proportion of wasting pigs, lack of response to therapy in affected individual accompanied by a high case fatality rate

Numbers of reported cases of PCVAD have increased rather dramatically in recent years. PCVAD now is widespread in the United States, Europe, and reported from most swine-producing areas. An apparent immune-mediated sequel to viral (perhaps PCV2) infection, porcine dermatopathy and nephropathy syndrome (PDNS) is sporadically reported. Circovirus is often associated with both PMWS and PDNS but PCV2 as sole cause remains in dispute. Other agents or risk factors are likely to be involved.

In utero infection with PCV2 may be inapparent, associated with reproductive failure or abortion. Because PCV2 is ubiquitous in swine populations and other agents or risk factors are frequently present, disease associations with PCV2 are sometimes difficult to prove.

Porcine circovirus Type 2 can contribute to PRDC in some herds. Experimental co-infection studies as well as anecdotal evidence suggests that PCV2 is likely to increase the severity of pneumonia caused *Mycoplasma hyopneumoniae*, swine influenza virus, porcine reproductive and respiratory syndrome virus (PRRS) and others.

Historical information

Since 1994, outbreaks of PMWS have been reported in North America and Europe and most swine-rearing areas of the world. The outbreaks have been consistently associated with PCV2 infection. Continued research and characterization of PCV2 remains of major interest among swine practitioners, researchers and producers. Genomic sequencing and restriction fragment length polymorphism (RFLP) techniques have defined several distinct viral clades within the PCV2 genotype but the clinical relevance of these distinctions is not completely understood.

Etiology

In 1982, a circovirus was isolated from porcine kidney cell line (PK-15) as an adventitious virus. Circoviruses are small, nonenveloped animal viruses with single-stranded circular DNA. Porcine circoviruses are quite hardy in the environment and in organic substrates. They are sensitive to most disinfectants but chlorhexidine, ethanol, and iodine are less effective. Circoviruses now are known to cause psittacine beak and feather disease, an infectious anemia in chickens, and lethal infections of pigeons, canaries and finches.

Two types of circoviruses in swine have been described. The PK-15 virus is referred to as Type I (PCV1). There is circumstantial evidence that PCV1 may be involved in congenital tremors but it is generally considered to be nonpathogenic for swine. Analysis has demonstrated that PCV associated with PCVAD in swine is distinctly different genetically and antigenically and it is now classified as PCV2. Antibodies between the two types have low cross-reactivity.

PCV2 is consistently present in pigs with PMWS, and disease has been reproduced by experimental infection with PCV2. Many but not all field cases of PCVAD have concurrent viral infections or some other evidence of immune stimulation that seems to allow permissive replication and pathologic effects of PCV2 in swine. Herds that are endemically infected with other significant pathogens, are operated on a continuous flow basis, are in swine dense areas, provide a suboptimal environment (air quality, hygiene), or practice poor biosecurity have been shown to be more likely to experience an outbreak of PCVAD. Once affected, these same herds often are presented with a more severe form of the disease.

Epidemiology

The epidemiology of porcine circovirus infections is speculative. Nearly all US swine herds are seropositive. Seroconversion usually occurs by two to four months of age irrespective of whether clinical signs of PCVAD are observed.

With PMWS, affected pigs are between two and four months of age and "waste away" while cohorts seem to grow normally. Morbidity varies from 2-30% but case fatality is high, approaching 80%. Transmission of the virus and conditions allowing virulence expression are being vigorously studied. Some risk factors purported include coinfection with other viruses (PRRSV, porcine parvovirus, etc.) or nonspecific immune stimulation (vaccination). Activated macrophages appear to be permissive for viral replication and persistence.

Pathogenesis

Pigs infected with PCV2 develop viremia of variable duration, with replication and persistence most extensive in macrophages and monocytes of lymphoid organs and lung. Lymphoid depletion at multiple sites, chronic lymphohistiocytic to granulomatous inflammation, and an erosive bronchiolitis with fibrosis are characteristic. Reproduction of typical lesions by inoculation with PCV2 has been inconsistent but there is general agreement among researchers that the virus is at least necessary and perhaps causal in order for PCVAD to be expressed. Mechanisms that allow disease expression and/ or immunity are not definitively known but appear to be related to macrophage activation prior to infection with PCV2. Occasionally, pigs may develop blotchy purple skin lesions and nephropathy, likely as an immune mediated sequel to viral infection, which is termed porcine dermatopathy and nephropathy syndrome (PDNS).

Clinical signs

PCVAD: Clinical signs include gradual wasting, unthriftiness, rough hair coat, polypnea, dyspnea, pallor, diarrhea, and occasionally icterus. To be defined as PCVAD, there must also be histologic lesions of lymphoid depletion and/or lymphohistiocytic to granulomatous inflammation in affected organs with PCV2 demonstrable within lesions. Affected pigs usually die; clinical survivors are severely stunted; non-clinical pigs in the same groups perform quite well. Both signs and lesions, as reported by various investigators, vary considerably.

PDNS: Is mainly a condition of pigs from 8-18 weeks of age. There are red-purple blotches on the skin, sometimes slightly raised, most obvious on the hind legs and perineum but can extend over the abdomen eventually covering the whole body. Most pigs with PDNS eventually die.

Lesions

PCVAD: Gross lesions include pallor, marked enlargement of all lymph nodes and perhaps spleen, and interstitial pattern of pneumonia in lungs. Less often present are icterus, a fluid-filled intestine, subcapsular white foci on the kidneys, atrophy of the liver and ulcers of the pars esophagea of the stomach. Microscopy reveals depletion of germinal centers in lymphoid tissues with replacement by histiocytes and multinucleated giant cells. Basophilic intracytoplasmic inclusion bodies often can be seen in macrophages in lymph nodes, tonsils, spleen and Peyer's patches. Lymphohistiocytic to granulomatous inflammation can be present in any organ, typically lungs and/or lymphoid tissues, and PCV2 antigen is abundantly present within characteristic lesions by immunohistochemistry (IHC) or in situ hybridization (ISH). Erosive bronchiolitis and fibrosis of airways is fairly typical.

PDNS: Often, there are small circumscribed circular to irregular, deep-purple discolorations of skin that become apparent on hind quarters, perineum, and flanks. Over the course of several days, the skin discolorations either resolve or expand and coalesce. Necropsy often reveals kidneys to be swollen with foci of pallor and/or hemorrhage in parenchyma. Microscopically, there is nonsuppurative vasculitis in sections of skin. Kidneys often have swollen glomerular tufts, inflammation, and protein in tubules. Multifocal nonsuppurative interstitial nephritis can also be a feature. The lesions are thought to be due to immune mediated (immune complex) vasculitis.

Lesions of PDNS are not specific for porcine circovirus.

Diagnosis

PCVAD: Diagnosis is made on clinical features, gross lesions, microscopic lesions, and demonstration of PCV2 within lesions. Using microscopy, characteristic lesions may be observed and virus inclusion bodies can often be identified in depleted lymph nodes, spleen, tonsils or Peyer's patches. Immunohistochemical tests or in situ hybridization are used to confirm diagnosis of disease associated with PCV2. Polymerase chain reaction (PCR) will confirm the presence of virus but does not confirm the presence of disease. Similarly, isolation and identification of a circovirus is not useful for diagnosis since asymptomatic infection is widespread in swine populations. Serological testing for both types of PCV has been developed to confirm infection but finding antibodies to circovirus in the herd is not diagnostic since most herds are positive without discernible disease. PCVAD must be differentiated from other bacterial or viral diseases, especially PRRSV which has similarities in clinical signs and lesion. Concurrent infections are common.

PDNS: Diagnosis of PDNS is by observing typical clinical signs, gross lesions, and histopathology. PCV2 antigen is demonstrable in some but not all cases.

Reproductive failure: In cases where reproductive failure is observed as abortions, stillbirths, and mummification, PCV2 can be demonstrated by IHC in fetal hearts as well as other tissues, in a routine diagnostic investigation.

Control

There is no specific treatment for pigs with PCVAD. However, anti-inflammatory agents and/or antimicrobials are sometimes used with some success in groups of pigs experiencing disease. All in/all out pig flow, thorough cleaning and disinfection between batches of pigs and early segregation and euthanasia of affected pigs are measures that may help control the disease. Antibiotics in feed or water may suppress secondary infections. Better definition of risk factors and intervention strategies for those factors may aid in control. Anecdotally, control of other infections (PRRSV, parvovirus, others) or altering timing of administration of vaccines has been of benefit in reducing the severity of PCVAD. Studies in Denmark have shown that that PCVAD can be eradicated from an affected farm by total depopulation. The ubiquitous nature of PCV2 makes it unlikely that commercial farms can be maintained free of the virus by this technique but relief from clinical effects of PCVAD can likely be achieved. Until the epidemiology, transmission, and virulence factors relating to PCV2 and PCVAD are further understood, use of total depopulation as a control strategy is not often recommended.

Porcine circovirus Type 2 has been identified in the semen of acutely affected boars. However, transmission of the virus (or PCVAD) via this route has not been documented in a field setting.

Porcine circovirus Type 2 vaccines became commercially available in the US in summer of 2006. Field experiences have demonstrated that the vaccines are effective in reducing the severity and incidence rate of PCVAD on many farms. The timing of vaccination and population to be immunized (breeding herds, replacement stock, growing pigs) varies between farms depending on the characteristics of the affected populations and the physical operation of the farm.

Porcine Picornaviruses (Enteroviruses)

Definition

A diverse group of diseases are caused by closely related viruses in the family Picornaviradae; the virus family has recently been reorganized. *Enterovirus* was one of seven genera in the family under the former taxonomy and contained numerous virus species to which swine were known to be susceptible, with virus species further designated by a serotyping scheme. Around 2000, the taxonomy was revised based on genomic sequence data. Currently, porcine enterovirus 1 (PEV 1, the prototype "Teschen virus" and "Talfan virus"), PEV 2 through 7, and PEV 11-13 have been moved to a new genus called *Teschovirus*. Porcine enteroviruses 8-10 remain in the original *Enterovirus* genus. Diseases manifested by the different viruses vary widely and include polioencephalomyelitis, female reproductive failure, myocarditis, pericarditis, pneumonia, and diarrhea.

Occurrence

Porcine picornaviruses are ubiquitous. They occur only in swine and most infections are asymptomatic. Teschen disease, the most virulent picornaviral infection, causes polioencephalomyelitis (PEM). The disease occurs only in central Europe and parts of Africa. Talfan disease, a similar but less severe disease, causes PEM in Europe, North America and Australia. Outbreaks in North America have occurred infrequently and been of minor significance.

Historical information

Teschen disease first was reported in Czechoslovakia over 65 years ago. Talfan disease was reported over 40 years ago. Both diseases, and other rather pathogenic picornaviral diseases, are well controlled and confined geographically and do not cause widespread problems in leading swine-raising countries. Other serogroups can occasionally cause polioencephalomyelitis outbreaks in the US.

Picornaviruses were once believed to be major causes of female reproductive failure and to cause stillbirths, mummification of fetuses, embryonic deaths and infertility (SMEDI). Although picornaviruses rarely can cause these abnormalities and occasional abortions, they are much less important than other known viral causes of reproductive failure. The picornaviruses are believed to cause other lesions or signs (including myocarditis, pericarditis, pneumonia and diarrhea), occur infrequently and seldom result in severe losses.

Etiology

There are more than 50 strains of porcine picornavirus. They can be grown readily in cell cultures of porcine origin. They are classified into 14 serogroups in the family Picornaviridae. Porcine enterovirus 1 (the prototype "Teschen virus" and "Talfan virus"), PEV 2 through 7, and PEV 11-13 have been moved to a new genus called *Teschovirus*. Porcine enteroviruses 8, 9 and 10 remain in the original *Enterovirus* genus. There is little cross reactivity among all these viruses. Picornaviruses are single-stranded RNA viruses, relatively stable, and highly resistant to environmental influences and many disinfectants. They can be inactivated by sodium hypochlorite.

Epidemiology

All picornaviruses are assumed to have similar epidemiology. Less virulent strains of virus are endemic in most herds. The viruses are shed in the feces and transmission usually is fecal-oral. Spread of virus usually is by direct or indirect contact with infected pigs. Infected fetuses born alive sometimes are a source of viral exposure of other pigs. Fomites can carry the relatively stable viruses. All ages of swine are susceptible if they have not previously encountered a picornavirus of that serogroup.

Pathogenesis

Picornavirus is ingested and replicates in the tonsil, intestinal tract and probably in lymphoid tissue in the lamina propria. The milder strains usually remain confined to the intestinal tract. Epithelial cell destruction is not a feature of picornaviral infections. With the more virulent strains, viremia occurs and virus may spread to the central nervous system (CNS) or pregnant uterus and fetuses.

Infections of the CNS vary in extent and severity and can affect that system from the olfactory bulbs to the lumbar cord. More often the lesions occur from the hypothalamus to the medulla. In prolonged cases there may be lymphocytic meningitis, particularly in the cerebellum and brain stem. Spinal cord lesions are largely confined to the gray matter of the ventral horns. There is a gradient in the severity of lesions and the outcome in an infected pig depends on location, severity and extent of lesions.

Clinical signs

Teschen disease, the most virulent porcine picornaviral infection, affects all age groups of swine. Morbidity and mortality are high. Early signs include anorexia, listlessness and fever which are soon followed by ataxia, abnormal postures and recumbency. There may be opisthotonus, convulsions, nystagmus and coma. Death occurs within a few days. Occasional cases survive but may have residual paralysis.

Talfan disease, a similar but less severe disease, results in lower morbidity and mortality. It usually occurs in young pigs, weaned or unweaned. Signs are similar to those of Teschen disease but milder. Although pigs often show ataxia and paresis, the paresis seldom progresses to paralysis and most pigs recover. Less virulent strains produce only mild or no CNS signs.

In the United States, occasional outbreaks of ataxia and posterior paresis are associated with other serogroups of picornavirus. Clinical signs are as described. Outbreaks are usually transient until herd immunity is established.

Lesions

There are no specific gross lesions caused by picornaviruses nor are there any microscopic lesions in the intestinal tract. In Teschen disease, Talfan disease and sporadic epidemics with the other newly classified viruses, there is a nonsuppurative inflammation prominent in the gray matter of the brain stem, cerebellum and spinal cord (polioencephalomyelitis). In affected areas many neurons are degenerate or necrotic. In prolonged cases there may be lymphocytic meningitis over the cerebellum and brain stem. Lesions tend to be more marked and extensive with Teschen disease than in cases caused by less virulent picornaviruses.

Diagnosis

Typical clinical signs and absence of gross lesions are suggestive of the diagnosis, especially in areas where outbreaks occurred previously. Microscopic lesions in the CNS are suggestive of viral infection but not pathognomonic. Paired serum samples taken at least two weeks apart may show a rising titer in serum neutralization or complement fixation tests. Virus isolation in tissue culture and identification by immunofluorescence or identification of viral antigen in tissue by similar technique are useful. These techniques are not available in all diagnostic laboratories in the United States since virulent porcine picornaviral infections seldom occur. Neurotropic picornaviral diseases must be differentiated from other diseases associated with CNS disease (see the table, Diseases Associated with CNS Signs, on page 152). Polymerase chain reaction (PCR) techniques have been widely reported and can helpful in both detection and identification of the virus. *Picornavirus* detected in nervous tissue should be considered diagnostic; when detected simply through serology or in enteric tissues further work should be completed in order to establish the significance of the virus. Many non-pathogenic strains can be routinely recovered from both normal and clinically ill pigs.

Control

In herds where picornaviruses have caused reproductive or other problems, new breeding stock should be introduced into the herd at least a month before breeding begins. They usually will be exposed to the endemic picornaviruses and develop an active immunity to them prior to breeding. It may be preferable to expose new stock to a composite sample of feces from the herd to which they are to be added. This can be done either by exposing them to pen contact with feces or mixing some feces with their feed.

In Europe, Teschen disease and Talfan disease have been controlled by slaughter and ring vaccination around premises or areas where outbreaks have occurred. Both live-attenuated and inactivated tissue culture vaccines have been used. In addition, there usually has been restriction of importations from endemic areas of infection.

In the US, occasional outbreaks of disease occur in nursery/grower stages. Most are transient but losses can be significant. Herd immunity is the goal but with segregation of ages, sometimes difficult to achieve.

Outbreaks of disease of unusual severity suspected of being caused by any of the virulent types of picornaviral infection should be reported immediately to livestock disease control authorities. Thus far, import regulations on swine and pork products have kept the United States free of most highly virulent porcine picornaviruses.

Porcine Reproductive and Respiratory Syndrome (PRRS)

Definition

PRRS is an acronym (porcine reproductive and respiratory syndrome) for a viral disease characterized by two overlapping clinical presentations, reproductive impairment or failure in breeding animals, and respiratory disease in pigs of any age. PRRS is the most economically significant disease to affect US swine production since the eradication of classical swine fever (CSF).

Occurrence

Porcine reproductive and respiratory syndrome virus (PRRSV) occurs in all age groups. Reproductive impairment or failure, more obvious in sows or gilts, also affects some boars. The respiratory syndrome is seen more often in young growing pigs but also occurs in naïve finishing pigs and breeding stock.

Although reported initially in only a few countries in the late 1980s, PRRS now occurs worldwide in most major swine-raising countries. PRRS is prevalent in the United States and exists both in epidemic and endemic forms.

Historical information

In the US, the clinical disease was first described in 1987-88 in North Carolina, Iowa and Minnesota. Several outbreaks in Indiana were reported in 1989-90. During the subsequent decade, PRRS spread rapidly, both in Europe and North America. By the end of 1992 the disease was reported in Canada, Great Britain and several European countries. Two distinct strains of virus, one in Europe and one in the United States, were characterized as genetically different but are clinically similar in most respects. Both are now in the United States, along with a multitude of viral variants.

The disease was first described as a syndrome and confused initially with several other diseases. It was referred to as swine mystery disease (SMD) or swine infertility and respiratory syndrome (SIRS) before porcine reproductive and respiratory syndrome (PRRS) became the generally agreed-upon name.

During the past 20 years, there has been much research on the PRRS virus. Although much now is known about the virus, details on control of the disease for all types of swine-raising operations are far from complete. PRRS is the most economically important disease now affecting producers. Swine industry consolidation of the past 15 years has led to entire production systems being designed around strategies for controlling or eliminating this disease.

Etiology

The PRRS virus is an enveloped RNA virus in the genus *Arterivirus*, classified in the virus family, *Arteriviridae*. There is considerable heterogeneity in the genome of the PRRS virus because of inherent errors common in transcription of RNA. The prototype US virus is related to but distinct from the first European isolate (referred to as Lelystad virus) identified in the Netherlands. There are significant genetic and antigenic differences between these initial isolates. Genetic and antigenic variability between isolates, even within a country, remains a continuous challenge to control of the disease.

The PRRS virus is only moderately resistant to environmental degradation. The virus is easily inactivated by phenol, formaldehyde, and most common disinfectants. The virus has a predilection for cells of the immune system, including pulmonary intravascular macrophages (PIM) and pulmonary alveolar macrophages (PAM); in the latter it replicates extensively. Primary PAMs and a limited number of continuous cell culture systems are used in isolating and maintaining virus. Strains of PRRS virus vary markedly in virulence. The basis for virulence differences is not yet known. Protective epitopes are not described nor can they be predicted from genomic analysis. The virus often appears to interact with other pathogenic viruses, bacteria and *Mycoplasma hyopneumoniae* to magnify severity of diseases.

Epidemiology

An important feature of the virus is its ability to persist in long-term carrier pigs (greater than 200 days). However, field observation suggests that most infected pigs eventually become immune, then cease to shed virus by 60 days post-infection. This is accompanied by a steady decline in antibody titers over a period of four to eight months after infection. Shedding carriers probably are the most common means of virus introduction to a herd or population of pigs. The virus is highly infectious (infectious dose is as little as 10 virions) but not highly contagious. It is present in nasal secretions, urine, semen, mammary secretions and feces. With the advent of artificial insemination, semen became a major source of viral introduction. The virus spreads readily by direct contact. There is limited experimental evidence of aerosol spread between farms but anecdotal opinions suggest it occurs at least sporadically. In some cases, infection is manifested as an epidemic of respiratory disease or reproductive failure but in other outbreaks, infection may spread slowly. Overall, virus transmission between groups of pigs is poorly understood. Debate continues as to roles of both vertical and/or lateral sources of infection in new outbreaks.

Sows infected while pregnant may deliver viremic, persistently infected piglets as a congenital PRRS virus infection. Virus can transmit from infected piglets or dams to other piglets. The cycle of shedding and infection can continue well into the nursery phase in situations where the sow herd is actively infected. Older infected pigs held back in nurseries or cross-fostered in the farrowing house often are a source of virus for younger pigs. Likewise, older pigs and their secretions can be a source of infection to younger pigs on premises where biosecurity between groups is lacking.

Boars are known to shed PRRS virus in semen for up to 92 days post-infection and can infect dams during breeding. Infection of sows occurs through natural breeding or artificial insemination. The advent of artificial insemination and boar studs has created a need for strict biosecurity and monitoring of PRRS virus in these facilities. Research suggests that the virus is unlikely to be spread to pigs by birds or rodents. There are no known replication-competent insect vectors but mosquitoes and house flies are capable of acting as fomites with the potential to spread the virus mechanically.

Pathogenesis

Once transmission of virus to the tonsil or upper respiratory system has occurred, primary replication occurs in lymphoid tissues. Viremia follows and may persist for several weeks. The virus has a predilection for lymphoid tissues (spleen, thymus, tonsils, lymph nodes, Peyer's patches). It infects and compromises the function of pulmonary alveolar and intravascular macrophages resulting in interstitial pneumonia. PRRS appears to increase susceptibility of the lungs to other pathogens.

PRRS virus is known to cross the placenta in late gestation (after the 72nd day) and may reach a high titer in fetuses. It may kill all, part or none of the fetuses. It is suggested that fetuses are killed by hypoxia that occurs as a result of the arteritis that may develop in umbilical vessels. Abortions are common, the result of either the effects of acute disease and fever in sows or infection and death of fetuses. Recovered sows are resistant to re-infection when exposed to a homologous strain of the virus but are likely to show clinical signs if a heterologous strain is encountered.

Clinical signs

PRRS is probably the most important swine disease of the last half-century. Serological testing has revealed there are many infected herds in which signs are not apparent. Where signs are apparent, they vary and are influenced by (1) virulence of the virus, (2) whether it is an initial infection or ongoing (endemic with herd immunity), (3) the age group affected, (4) other disease causing agents present in the population, and (5) herd size and management practices.

Breeding age gilts, sows, and boars: Clinical signs may include a period of anorexia, fever, lethargy, depression, and perhaps respiratory distress or vomiting. Mild cyanosis of the ears, abdomen and vulva has been reported in some outbreaks. Reproductive problems, often the most obvious signs, include a decrease in the number of dams that conceive or farrow. There is usually an increase in premature farrowings, late term abortions, stillborn or weak piglets and mummified fetuses. Preweaning mortality is high. Nursing pigs may have dyspnea ("thumping"). The period for reproductive signs varies with herd size but is usually two to three months in duration. A slow improvement in reproductive performance then begins. In larger operations, signs may be cyclical, especially if naïve gilts or sows continue to be introduced into the herd. There is evidence that subpopulations within large breeding herds escape initial infection but are infected when exposed later and serve as sources of continued virus shedding. Also, herds may be infected with multiple, heterologous strains of PRRS virus that are not completely cross-protective. In boars, clinical signs are similar to sows and are accompanied by a decrease in semen quality.

Young, growing and finishing pigs: Primary clinical signs among young pigs are fever, depression, lethargy, stunting due to systemic disease, and pneumonia. Sneezing, fever and lethargy are followed by expiratory dyspnea and stunting. Peak age for respiratory disease is four to ten weeks. Postweaning mortality often is markedly increased, especially with more virulent strains and the occurrence of ever-present concurrent and secondary infections. Older pigs, especially naïve, high-health swine, have similar respiratory signs. Heterologous infections may lead to prolonged or repeated outbreaks of respiratory disease.

Lesions

PRRS virus infection generally results in mild to severe lesions in lungs and lymph nodes. The interstitial pneumonia varies from multifocal to lobular to diffuse in distribution. Lungs appear mottled and tan but are highly variable in extent. Lymph nodes are generally swollen, tan and edematous or cystic. Microscopic lesions may include nonsuppurative interstitial pneumonia, mild nonsuppurative encephalitis, myocarditis, rhinitis, and perhaps depletion of germinal centers of lymph nodes.

Most fetuses and stillborn pigs with uncomplicated PRRS have no discernible lesions but some may have umbilical cord arteritis and hemorrhage; patchy distribution of slightly firm lungs (interstitial pneumonia); enlargement of lymph nodes; hemorrhages in the skin; edema of the eyelids, periorbital tissues, colonic mesentery and various body cavities; and dehydration with prominence of the vertebral column. Sows with acute PRRS virus infection have typical lung and systemic lesions. Endometritis, myometritis and placental lesions have been reported.

Other infections are common in pigs with PRRS. Differential diagnosis for respiratory disease includes lesions or co-infections caused by influenza virus, *Streptococcus suis*, *Mycoplasma hyopneumoniae*, *Salmonella choleraesuis*, *Haemophilus parasuis*, *Pasteurella multocida*, porcine circovirus, porcine respiratory coronavirus, and *Actinobacillus pleuropneumoniae*.

Diagnosis

Clinical signs and history often suggest PRRS, especially in acute outbreaks. Characteristic microscopic lesions in lungs and several other tissues also are suggestive but not pathognomonic. PRRS infection is widespread in US herds so care must be taken to both confirm an active infection and to rule out other infectious diseases. Any tentative clinical diagnosis should be confirmed by detection of the PRRS virus. This can be by virus isolation (VI), detection of PRRS antigen by fluorescent antibody tests (FAT) or immunohistochemistry (IHC), or detection of PRRS virus genome by polymerase chain reaction (PCR) and be coupled with presence of typical lesions. Serology provides indirect evidence of infection but does not determine if there is actual disease caused by PRRS virus.

Detection of PRRS virus is best performed in affected pigs during the early stages of PRRS infection. Suitable specimens are obtained from weak-born neonates that have not nursed, or clinically affected (thumping, febrile) nursing pigs, and from febrile, anorectic postweaned pigs and sows. Probably the best tissues for virus detection methods include bronchoalveolar lavage (BAL), serum, lung, lymph nodes, tonsil and spleen.

Aborted, mummified, or stillborn pigs are sometimes (50% positive) useful for diagnosis by performing PCR on fluids and also for ruling out other infections. Sows that are not sick at the time of abortion are usually not viremic but should have high antibody levels in serum. Sows that are acutely ill should have virus in serum that can be detected by PCR or virus isolation.

Viral antigen can be identified in infected fresh tissue, preferably lung, by direct fluorescent antibody test but is more commonly identified in formalin fixed tonsil or lung by IHC. Using IHC, the virus can be visualized within typical lesions. PCR or in situ hybridization can be used to demonstrate viral RNA.

Serology may be helpful in confirming the presence (seropositivity) and stage (high levels of antibody in recent infections) of PRRS infection in the herd. A series of blood samples from various stages of production is useful to determine the age that PRRSV is most commonly infecting pigs. Several different tests for PRRS antibody have been used. In the United States, indirect immunofluorescent antibody (IFA), serum neutralization, and enzyme-linked immunosorbent assay (ELISA) tests often are used. ELISA has many advantages, including automation, an approximate quantification of antibody, and the ability to identify both European and American strains of virus. Finding PRRS virus antibodies in a few serum samples may not be evidence of active disease; many "normal" herds have animals with antibodies and maternally derived antibody may be detectable up to six weeks of age.

Techniques for differentiating viral isolates are sometimes available, including the use of restriction enzymes and RNA fragment analysis (RFLP) or actual sequencing of portions of the viral genome. Thus far, sequencing has been a valuable epidemiology tool but neither it nor RFLP predict antigenicity or the presence of cross-protective epitopes. The value of sequencing is determining the relatedness (homology) of two or more PRRS virus isolates to determine source of infection or whether more than one "strain" is present in a population.

Control

There is no single successful strategy for control of PRRS, largely because of virus variation, large swine populations, and unresolved issues of transmission. In some smaller herds, immunity may be sufficient so that infection is not causing significant economic losses, in which case no intervention is necessary. Often, there are sufficient losses to consider some or all of the following points for control. A control program should be tailored to fit the individual farm situation.

An accurate diagnosis is essential to confirm the disease and epidemiology on a particular farm. This requires both disease characterization (demonstrate disease agents and lesions) and a serologic profile of pigs in the various stages of production. Serologic testing of a significant sample of animals from each stage of production should indicate the stage (acute or chronic) of infection in the herd as well where and how the virus is being spread in the herd. Once the disease is defined, a strategy can be developed to achieve one of two general goals, either to eliminate PRRS or to control ("live with") PRRS.

The goal of many herds is to "stabilize" the infection in the sow herd by assuring immunity in all breeding stock. This "herd immunity" prevents the reproductive failure and can decrease the likelihood of transmission of virus from dams to fetuses and offspring. When coupled with segregated rearing of offspring, clinical effects of infection can be minimized. Breeding herd stabilization can sometimes be accomplished by vaccination, intentional whole-herd infection, aggressive acclimatization of replacement breeding stock, or combinations of these strategies.

Two major, generally recognized as essential, components are to limit the frequency of seed stock introductions to the sow herd and to assure that the replacement gilts be well-acclimatized to the PRRS virus present in the sow herd. Seed stock introductions to sow herds should not be more frequent than monthly, with quarterly or semiannual introductions preferred. Assuring infection of replacement gilts, followed by at least 60 days recovery (cool-down) before they enter the sow herd is strongly recommended. Ideally, replacement gilts should originate from a single, PRRS-negative source and be infected only with the PRRS strain(s) present in a particular sow herd.

Boars introduced into negative herds should be quarantined for 60-90 days after purchase and confirmed negative serologically. Those entering PRRS-positive herds require acclimatization to resident PRRS virus in a fashion similar to gilts. Many organizations that provide semen for artificial insemination now use PCR to assure that semen is free of PRRS virus.

Sow herds and offspring that remain positive for PRRS may prefer to strive for minimizing clinical effect rather than trying to eradicate it and prevent re-infection. Acclimatization of breeding animals and management of pig flow allows for some success in "living with" PRRS. There are both killed and live commercial vaccines for control of reproductive and/or respiratory forms of PRRS that may be useful; experience suggests they are inconsistently efficacious. Autogenous killed PRRS vaccines have also been used with very limited success.

Herds successfully "stabilized" for PRRS virus may produce PRRS-negative offspring. Once the breeding herd is producing PRRS-negative offspring, it is necessary to evaluate the nursery, grower and finisher phases. Initial testing should indicate whether it would be necessary to depopulate, clean and disinfect these stages. Nursery depopulation often improves production. All phases of production should use all in/all out management.

Some sow herds that consistently produce negative offspring may attempt to eliminate PRRS from the sow herd. At that point, all subsequent replacement seed stock should be naïve for PRRS infection and any residual infected sows in the herd should be eliminated. The latter has been accomplished by testing (serology, PCR) and removal, or in some cases, by normal attrition.

In some operations, it may be economically feasible to depopulate, clean and disinfect the facilities and, after a few weeks, repopulate with stock free of PRRS and other major diseases. Herd closure for at least 200 days has also been used as another means to stabilize a breeding herd without having to depopulate. Most breeding stock companies today provide PRRS-free seed stock which was once a major limitation. Before embarking on this strategy, one should honestly assess risk factors for re-infection of the herd as well as the level of biosecurity that can be maintained by the producer. Herds located in swine-dense areas are at great risk for re-infection.

There is no specific treatment for PRRS. Broad-spectrum antibiotics may be useful in controlling secondary infections. Anti-inflammatory products (e.g. aspirin) are commonly administered during acute disease. Other helpful techniques include early weaning and isolation of piglets, various PRRS vaccination protocols, regular serologic monitoring, testing (ELISA, PCR and IFA) and removal of persistent carriers in herds with <10% infection, and improving biosecurity.

Since the PRRS virus, the control strategies, and the specific farm situations are so variable, it is imperative that experienced practitioners, diagnosticians and research workers continue to objectively expand their knowledge to better control and eventually eliminate this financially devastating disease.

Pox (Swine Pox)

Definition

A viral disease that is characterized by the acute appearance of round to oval cutaneous lesions that heal in three to four weeks.

Occurrence

Swine pox occurs only in swine. All age groups are susceptible but most outbreaks are encountered in young growing pigs. It occasionally occurs congenitally and in neonates. Swine pox occurs worldwide in the major swine-raising countries. It occurs more often where insect vectors of pox virus are not controlled. Modern swine raised free of lice rarely exhibit the disease.

Historical information

Swine pox was first reported in Europe in 1842 and in the United States in 1929. The disease persisted and was relatively common, perhaps because it caused little obvious economic loss to swine producers. Outbreaks once were caused by two viruses: vaccinia virus, a laboratory strain, and swine pox virus. Vaccinia virus is no longer used to vaccinate people against small pox; hence it no longer spreads to pigs. Only swine pox virus now causes pox in swine.

Etiology

Swine pox virus, a member of the Poxviridae family, is the etiologic agent. The virus is rather resistant to environmental degradation; it persists in scabs for up to a year. Microscopically, the virus is visible as large intracytoplasmic inclusions in infected cells.

Epidemiology

Persistent virus within desquamated scabs can be transmitted to other pigs when introduced into skin abrasions. The virus can also spread horizontally from nasal and oral secretions from infected pigs. Once a few virus-containing lesions appear, the virus can be transmitted mechanically by the bites of vectors that have recently fed in pox lesion areas. Common vectors include the hog louse (*Haematopinus suis*), mosquitoes, and biting flies. Once introduced, infected swine or virus-carrying biting insects can initiate outbreaks in susceptible herds. There is evidence of transplacental infection of neonatal pigs.

Pathogenesis

Virus introduced into abrasions replicates in cells of the stratum spinosum causing typical skin lesions to develop. The lesions go through the stages of macules, papules, vesicles, pustules and crusts. All but the vesicle stage are easily identified. As lesions mature and heal, crusts containing virus desquamate and leave white macules.

A viremic stage of the disease has not been demonstrated. However, it must occur in some animals since transplacental infection of neonatal piglets has been reported. Antibody to pox virus is formed as a consequence of infection and immunity is long lasting.

Clinical signs and lesions

Systemic clinical signs of disease seldom are observed but the skin lesions are easily seen. Initial lesions usually are along the ventral aspect of the abdomen, inside the legs and in inguinal areas, all favorite feeding sites of hog lice. However, lesions have been observed at many cutaneous sites so most of the skin appears susceptible. Initially, there are small vesicles that largely are unnoticed. The papules that result are seen as 1-3 mm circular red spots. As lesions mature, crusts form that eventually heal uneventfully. In severe infections, lesions may occur in upper respiratory and digestive tracts. This is particularly true of congenitally-acquired pox where piglets are born with or develop lesions over the entire body shortly after birth. Exudative epidermitis (greasy pig disease) and secondary bacterial dermatitis occasionally occur as a sequel to swine pox. Swine pox does not appear to cause a pruritic response in affected pigs.

Diagnosis

Swine pox is easily diagnosed by identifying the lesions. Lesions are round to oval, usually less than 1.0 cm in diameter. The brown to black crusts are easily seen but the vesicle stage seldom can be identified grossly. If confirmation is needed, histologic diagnosis can be made by identifying typical, large, intracytoplasmic inclusion bodies in cutaneous lesions. Pox lesions should be differentiated from those of other vesiculating viral diseases, pityriasis rosea, dermatosis vegetans, streptococcal dermatitis, ringworm and greasy pig disease.

Control

Control of swine pox relies on herd immunity and prevention of transmission. Pox seldom is a problem if the usual vectors of virus, especially hog lice, are controlled by insecticides or elimination. Congenital swine pox is generally a sporadic, self-limiting event. There are no treatments.

Pseudorabies (Aujeszky's Disease)

Definition

Pseudorabies (PRV) is a major viral disease manifested in swine by signs and lesions that vary among different age groups. The disease is characterized by three overlapping syndromes that reflect lesions in the central nervous system (CNS), respiratory system or reproductive system.

Occurrence

Among domestic animals, swine are the only natural host of pseudorabies virus (PRV). All age groups not previously exposed or vaccinated are susceptible. The disease was eradicated from the US commercial pig industry in 2004 but remains in some localized feral swine populations. The disease remains common in many other major swine-raising countries. Most domestic animals (cattle, sheep, dogs, cats, and goats but not horses) and many wild animals (rats, mice, raccoons, opossums, rabbits, and several fur-bearing mammals) are susceptible to the virus but transmission only occurs when these species are kept in close contact with acutely infected swine; death is the usual outcome in these aberrant hosts. Pseudorabies occurs with some frequency in both cattle and sheep, especially those in close contact with swine. There is no evidence that PRV is a health threat to humans.

Historical information

The disease is named after the Hungarian veterinarian Dr. Aladár Aujeszky who linked the disease in cattle, dogs, and cats in 1902. Pseudorabies was not identified as a viral disease in swine until 1909.

Prior to 1960, the disease in swine was important in Eastern Europe but major outbreaks did not occur in the US until the mid-1970s. Incidence of the disease increased with the widespread introduction of total confinement and continuous farrowing during this period. Additionally, antiserum used in control of classical swine fever prior to this period often contained antibodies to PRV and likely contributed to suppression of clinical signs on many farms. Active PRV eradication programs exist in many countries and have been successful, in large part due to efficacious differential vaccination.

In 1989, the US embarked on a 5-stage Federal/State/Industry program for eradication of PRV in swine; eradication of PRV from the commercial industry was achieved in 2004.

Etiology

Pseudorabies virus (PRV) is an alphavirus in a subfamily of Herpesviridae. Isolates vary in virulence and pathogenicity. Like many other herpesviruses, PRV often persists in a latent state in recovered animals. The virus is only moderately resistant outside the host, survival depending largely on environmental factors. Except during cold weather, virus probably does not survive more than two weeks outside the pig. Under exceptional conditions it may survive longer in infected fetuses, dried tissue, and buildings. The virus can be destroyed by many disinfectants, including orthophenylphenol, quarternary ammonium or iodine compounds, and 5% sodium hydroxide.

At least nine proteins, many of them structural proteins on the virus envelope, have been identified. By genetic engineering it has been possible to prepare effective vaccines that omit one or more of the proteins. Antibodies to such vaccines differ sufficiently from antibodies to wild virus so that serologic tests can identify naturally infected herds. Protection induced by commercial PRV vaccines appears to be effective against all wild types of the virus.

Epidemiology

Pseudorabies virus is spread and persists by several mechanisms. Swine that recover from PRV excrete large amounts of virus in saliva and nasal secretions, and perhaps in urine and feces, for up to two weeks. Virus can persist in the tonsils of carrier swine for at least several weeks. Latent virus can persist in the CNS for many months. Recrudescence and shedding of virus often occur after stress.

Inapparent shedders frequently are the means of introduction of virus into susceptible herds. Once introduced, the virus spreads by nose-to-nose contact, through feed and water contaminated by oral secretions and by aerosols coughed into the air. Circumstantial evidence suggests that an infectious aerosol can spread several miles.

In a farrowing house, aborted fetuses or infected piglets born alive or incubating the disease soon contaminate the house. Virus may survive long enough to infect piglets of the next farrowing.

Feral swine remain a possible source of infection to domestic swine. Other PRV-infected animals (e.g. rats, mice, dogs, cats, raccoons, opossums) are considered "dead-end" hosts and will shed PRV only a short time. They may, however, visit swine facilities and either shed virus that contaminates the facility or they may die and be eaten by swine. The possible role of flies or birds in transmission is dubious.

Pathogenesis

Pathogenesis is variable, depending on virulence of the viral strain, age of the pig and the route and severity of exposure. Experimentally, pigs can be infected by many routes of inoculation. Under field conditions the oral-nasal routes of exposure probably are most common. Virus often localizes in epithelium of the tonsils. The primary site of replication is epithelium of tonsils and nasopharynx. With highly virulent strains of virus there may be a short period of viremia with dissemination to many tissues. Most viral strains have a tropism for the CNS and upper respiratory tract.

The virus also can spread from a primary site of infection along nerves to the CNS, then to the spinal cord and spread centrifugally along nerve trunks. Virus often localizes in ganglia, e.g. the trigeminal nerve ganglia and paravertebral ganglia, and may become latent there. It may be reactivated later by stress.

In many areas of localization, including respiratory epithelium, the virus causes inflammation and necrosis of tissue. In some organs and tissues, necrotic areas often are large enough to be grossly visible. Virus may cross the placenta to infect some or all fetuses. In the reproductive tract, the virus causes endometritis, vaginitis, and necrotic placentitis. Lesions and virus may be present in infected fetuses. Intranuclear inclusion bodies are produced in a variety of cells in swine of all ages, including fetuses.

Clinical signs

Signs vary, depending largely on the immune status of the dam and the age of the pigs affected. In general, younger pigs are more severely affected but become more resistant as they age. Neonatal pigs born to naïve sows are highly susceptible to infection and piglets become ill two to four days after exposure. Very young neonates may die without signs even having been noticed. Nursing pigs usually show signs of neurologic involvement. Signs may include high fever, depression, anorexia, tremors, incoordination, dog-sitting position, vomiting, foaming at the mouth, blindness, paddling, coma and convulsions. Death often occurs within one to three days. Morbidity and mortality may approach 100% in neonates, especially in naïve herds. Piglets nursing recovered or vaccinated dams are well protected from clinical signs and infection with the virus.

Weaned pigs (three to nine weeks of age) have similar signs but mortality is usually much lower. Respiratory signs often occur in the older pigs of this age group. They include sneezing, nasal discharge, sometimes coughing and labored breathing. Most of the pigs survive, provided they do not succumb to secondary infections, especially bacterial pneumonia.

In susceptible, grow/finish swine (ten weeks of age to market weight), respiratory signs predominate and morbidity is high. Signs include a febrile response, depression, anorexia, sneezing, coughing and nasal discharge. CNS signs occur in occasional pigs and vary in severity from tremors to convulsions. Most pigs recover in about seven to ten days.

In breeding herds, clinical signs may not be apparent except during the period of initial infection. These signs are primarily respiratory and most animals will recover. In pregnant sows or gilts, reproductive failure sometimes occurs. Dams infected in the first trimester may absorb their fetuses and return to estrus. Those in the second or third trimester may abort or have mummified, stillborn or weak pigs. Those infected close to term may deliver infected piglets that die within a few days. Reproductive failure usually has a modest incidence of < 20%.

Lesions

Neonates that die acutely after infection may have no gross lesions. In piglets showing CNS signs, congestion of the meninges often is visible. In those showing respiratory signs, there may be a rhinitis with patchy epithelial necrosis. The rhinitis can be seen after splitting the skull and nasal bones midsagittally. The inflammation often extends into the fauces and larynx, and occasionally into the trachea or esophagus. Other gross lesions may include keratoconjunctivitis and necrosis of the tonsils. Gross and/or microscopic foci of necrosis may be seen in the liver, spleen, lungs, adrenals and lymph nodes. Similar foci sometimes are present in aborted fetuses.

Microscopic lesions often include a panencephalitis, ganglioneuritis at multiple sites, and perhaps nonsuppurative meningitis. The most severe lesions in the brain usually are in the cerebral cortex and often include neuronal degeneration and necrosis. In the lungs there may be bronchitis, bronchiolitis and alveolitis with hemorrhagic foci of necrosis but lung lesions generally are neither severe nor specific. Intranuclear inclusion bodies may be found at many sites, often within neurons, astrocytes, oligodendroglia and respiratory epithelium. They are more easily demonstrated in mercury-fixed tissues.

In dams that have infected fetuses or abort, the uterine wall may be thickened by inflammatory edema. Necrotic placentitis may be apparent in the placenta of infected fetuses and neonatal piglets.

Diagnosis

Diagnosis often can be made on the basis of prevalence of the disease in the area, history, signs, gross and microscopic lesions or serologic testing. Serologic tests available include serum neutralization (SN), latex agglutination (LA), and enzyme-linked immunosorbent assay (ELISA). SN is the standard regulatory test but the LA and ELISA tests are widely used as screening tests. Serologic testing is widely used for herd diagnosis. Accurate serologic tests that can differentiate vaccination antibody from wild type are widely available and are commonly used as part of national disease control programs. A fluorescent antibody test on tissue sections, immunohistochemistry on formalin-fixed tissues, or virus isolation may be used to identify virus in the brain, tonsils, and spleen. A polymerase chain reaction (PCR) test has been described but is not in common use.

Control

Pseudorabies is currently considered an exotic viral disease in the US since its eradication in 2004. In countries where the disease remains endemic, it may be possible to prevent exposure of a negative herd to PRV through strict quarantine and isolation procedures. Only seronegative animals should be added, as necessary, to a herd. Additions should be made only after a quarantine period of at least one month and negative serologic tests before and after quarantine. Cats, dogs, rats, mice and all wildlife should be prevented from coming in contact with swine.

An all in/all out system with cleaning and disinfection between farrowings is helpful. Gene-deleted modified-live vaccines are available and their use is accompanied by the application of ELISA serologic tests that can differentiate infected from vaccinated swine. These vaccines are safe and concerns about return to virulence have been effectively dismissed. Pseudorabies vaccines increase resistance to PRV infection, virtually eliminate clinical signs associated with infection, and minimize the amount of viral shedding that results if infection occurs. The incidence of latency and frequency of recrudescence of virus in latently infected swine are also decreased in vaccinated swine.

There is no effective treatment for PRV-infected swine but weaned and older swine often recover.

Rotaviral Enteritis

Definition

Rotaviruses cause diarrhea in nursing and postweaned pigs, affecting primarily the small intestine. If uncomplicated, diarrhea is accompanied by high morbidity and low mortality.

Occurrence

Rotaviruses are ubiquitous in swine populations throughout the world. Rotavirus infections occur in many species, including man. Although rotaviruses are related antigenically, porcine rotaviruses infect only swine.

Historical information

In 1969, rotaviruses were identified in calves. Subsequently, they were detected in other animals, including swine and humans. Rotaviral infections are important because they are common and reduce productivity.

Etiology

There are at least 7 antigenically distinct serogroups of rotaviruses (A, B, C, D, E, F, G) of which 4 (A, B, C, E) affect swine. There are also antigenically dissimilar subgroups or serovarieties within groups. Most is known about the more common group A rotaviruses. Group A is by far the most prevalent but type C has been associated with outbreaks. Immunity is not cross-protective between serogroups and is incomplete between serovarieties.

Rotaviruses are very stable in the environment. They are resistant to temperature changes, many chemicals, various pH levels, and many disinfectants. Recommended disinfectants for cleaned surfaces include formaldehyde and chlorine-based disinfectants including chlorox.

Epidemiology

It is likely that all large swine herds are infected and rotaviruses circulate constantly in them. Neonatal and susceptible young growing pigs are exposed to virus shed by carriers, including sows, or that is present in their environment. They may develop clinical or subclinical disease but most pigs recover with at least some becoming carriers. The resistance of rotaviruses in the environment assures their survival on swine-raising premises during short periods of depopulation. The possibility of interspecies spread of rotaviruses has not been studied extensively.

Rotaviral infection can occur concurrently with other diarrheal diseases of young pigs, e.g. with transmissible gastroenteritis, colibacillosis, or salmonellosis. Combined infections with other agents cause more severe clinical signs and lead to higher mortality.

Pathogenesis

The pathogenesis of type A rotaviral infection in pigs is much the same as for transmissible gastroenteritis (TGE). Exposure to virus is fecal-oral. The virus is swallowed and reaches the small intestine. Virus invades intestinal epithelial cells on the tips of the villi and damages or destroys many of them. The result is villous atrophy with fusion of some villi. Villous destruction can be subtle, segmental, or severe but generally is less severe than with TGE.

Destruction of villous epithelium and villous fusion result in impaired intestinal function and reduced disaccharidase activity. Disaccharides accumulate in the intestine. An osmotic movement of fluid into the intestinal lumen, along with malabsorption, leads to diarrhea. Death is an unusual outcome but probably is related to multiple factors including malnutrition, dehydration, imbalance of electrolytes and cardiac failure. The pathogenesis of types B, C and E rotaviral infections are likely similar to that of type A.

Clinical signs

The onset and severity of signs depends on dose ingested and amount of protective antibody in the dam's colostrum and milk. Outbreaks on specific premises often occur repeatedly when the piglets reach an age at which lactogenic immunity is no longer adequate to protect against the degree of exposure.

Diarrhea appears, usually white to yellow in color, and generally continues for a few days until the pigs develop an active immunity. There is moderate dehydration. Vomiting occurs but is not a major clinical sign. Morbidity is variable but mortality usually is low or none when good housing and husbandry is present. Signs, morbidity and mortality are enhanced if there is concurrent disease, poor husbandry or exposure to cold.

Lesions

Pigs that die are dehydrated and may show fecal staining of the perineal area. The intestinal wall is thin, flaccid and rather transparent. The small intestine and colon contain yellow or gray fluid and debris. Microscopic lesions are largely confined to villi of the terminal jejunum and ileum; the duodenum is not spared as with TGE. Microscopy reveals villous atrophy with some fusion of villi as well as epithelial hyperplasia in crypts.

Necrosis of apical enterocytes is followed by squamous and cuboidal metaplasia as lesions resolve.

Diagnosis

History, signs and gross lesions are helpful but not diagnostic. A variety of laboratory techniques are available to establish a firm diagnosis. Electron microscopy can be used to identify virions in the intestinal content or viral particles in affected epithelial cells. Fluorescent antibody technique and immunohistochemistry can demonstrate rotavirus in the epithelial cells. Using light microscopy, the typical lesions of villous atrophy and glandular hyperplasia may be useful in diagnosis. Rotaviral antigens in fresh fecal samples or intestinal fluid sometimes can be detected using an enzyme-linked immunosorbent assay (ELISA) test.

Virus shedding is much greater during early stages of the disease so samples should be obtained from acutely affected pigs.

Control

There are no proven specific therapies for rotaviral infection in young piglets. However, good husbandry and supportive therapy, including electrolytes in drinking water, can be of value. A dry, warm environment and good nutrition are important in reducing severity of outbreaks. Antibiotics are not effective for rotaviral infections but may be indicated for concurrent bacterial diseases.

The all in/all out system with thorough cleaning and disinfection between farrowings and a high standard of sanitation reduces exposure of piglets to rotavirus. A shorter farrowing period is less likely to lead to a build up of rotaviruses in the farrowing house. Similarly, all in/all out population of nurseries will decrease the dose and lessen the effects of rotavirus infections postweaning. Rotavirus as a consistent cause of diarrhea in post-weaned pigs would implicate poor sanitation, and disinfecting between groups of pigs would be warranted. Decreasing dose by scrupulous sanitation is high priority for breaking the cycle of disease.

Both modified live virus and killed rotavirus vaccines are available. Dams can be vaccinated at intervals prior to farrowing to stimulate them to produce antibody in their colostrum and milk. The antibody should protect their piglets until piglets have time to develop their own immunity. Booster vaccinations are given before subsequent farrowings, sometimes after farrowing. Alternatively, some swine raisers intentionally expose their new breeding stock to resident stock, or to their feces, prior to breeding. In this way added stock will develop immunity to indigenous rotaviruses being shed by older stock. Most rotavirus vaccines are combined with vaccines for control of other diarrheal diseases. Most are made to control only type A rotaviral infection.

Transmissible Gastroenteritis (TGE)

Definition
Transmissible gastroenteritis (TGE) is an acute, rapidly spreading, viral disease of swine of all ages, characterized by diarrhea and vomiting. High mortality in piglets under two weeks of age is common with mortality decreasing with age. There also is an endemic form of the disease, seen in herds with partial immunity or concurrent porcine respiratory coronavirus (PRCV) infection, with less severe signs and much lower mortality.

Occurrence
Transmissible gastroenteritis (TGE) occurs naturally only in swine. Among previously unexposed swine, all age groups are susceptible. TGE occurs throughout the year but incidence may be higher in the colder months. TGE occurs in many major swine-raising countries but is seen infrequently in Europe.

Historical information
In the United States, outbreaks that were likely TGE were seen as early as 1943 but the first documented outbreaks were reported in 1946. Subsequently, the disease was identified in many other countries.

Serologic surveys indicate that TGE is widespread throughout the US. Although initial outbreaks are acute, a less severe, endemic form now persists in some herds. TGE can cause up to 100% neonatal mortality during the initial stages of an outbreak and is therefore unlikely to be misdiagnosed in a previously naïve herd.

In Europe, and more recently in the US, TGE is seldom seen because a natural mutant of TGE virus, porcine respiratory coronavirus (PRCV) presumably stimulates immunity to TGE.

Etiology
The etiologic agent of TGE is a coronavirus (TGEV). Most isolates are enteropathic. Virus is labile at about 72° F (22° C), but quite stable when frozen. A closely related virus, porcine respiratory coronavirus (PRCV), is present in many countries, including the United States. Canine coronavirus and feline infectious peritonitis viruses are related to TGEV.

The PRCV is derived from TGEV by deletion of the S-gene. It has lost its tropism for enterocytes but has increased tropism for the lungs. It can cause a mild respiratory disease in swine although most infections are subclinical. Serologically, TGEV and PRCV cross-react but tests are available to distinguish between them. TGEV can be destroyed by many disinfectants, e.g. iodides, quaternary ammonium compounds, phenol and sodium hypochlorite.

Epidemiology
Swine that survive TGE develop antibodies against the virus but continue to excrete virus in their feces or nasal secretions for at least two to eight weeks; some individuals have been shown to excrete virus intermittently for up to 18 months. TGE virus has been isolated from intestinal and lung homogenates for up to 104 days. Infected sows can transmit virus in their milk or feces to their piglets. Although feces are the major source of infection, virus probably is spread aerogenously, at least for short distances. In feeding operations or multiple farrowing operations, where animals from multiple sources are intermixed, carrier animals often are a source of exposure to TGE virus. Other animals and insects known to act as mechanical carriers of virus for various lengths of time and distance include dogs, cats, foxes, starlings and flies.

The virus is resistant enough that fomites readily transmit the virus. Once introduced, virus may persist on premises, especially during the colder months. Conversely, premises depopulated for a few days during hot summer months may then be free of virus.

When virus is introduced into a herd of naïve swine, all age groups are affected and the disease assumes epidemic characteristics. Once premises are infected and there is a constant source of immunologically naïve pigs because of frequent or continuous farrowing or frequent introduction of susceptible animals, TGE may persist as a chronic disease in the herd. Infection often persists in successive groups of pigs entering a contaminated nursery.

Factors other than virulence of the virus and host resistance seem to play little part in susceptibility to infection. Outbreaks often occur on premises with excellent husbandry, nutrition and sanitation.

Pathogenesis
The virus enters the pharynx via the oral or nasal route, is swallowed and reaches susceptible epithelial cells of the small intestine. In neonates or young pigs, infection of those cells with destruction or loss of function is accompanied by patchy atrophy of intestinal villi most noticeable in the jejunum and ileum. The lesions lead to malabsorption of nutrients. Inability to hydrolyze lactose in dam's milk leads to an osmotic flow of fluids into the intestinal lumen. This results in diarrhea and dehydration. Death is related to dehydration, metabolic acidosis and abnormal cardiac function caused by hyperkalemia. In very young pigs, the relatively high proportion of absorptive enterocytes and the relatively slow regeneration time of epithelial cells to cover denuded villi, coupled with the limited ability to maintain homeostasis, results in very high mortality.

Clinical signs
In acute outbreaks, the incubation period is very short, 18 hrs to three days. In baby pigs the disease spreads rapidly to affect all susceptible pigs. Signs include profuse diarrhea, frequent vomiting, rapid dehydration, shivering and marked thirst. The pigs weaken rapidly and usually die within one to two days. Pigs suckling immune dams may remain well as long as they receive adequate antibody in the dam's colostrum and milk. Pigs infected after 4 weeks of age often survive.

The chronic or endemic form of TGE often is seen in pigs from herds where some dams are immune and others have a limited immunity. Onset of clinical signs varies, depending on when lactogenic immunity fails and leaves them susceptible, but is usually later in lactation or early in the postweaning period (two to five weeks of age). Signs can be rather mild, especially in well-doing pigs, and usually include diarrhea, dehydration, unthriftiness and runting.

In feeder and fattening pigs, signs usually are mild except for diarrhea which is profuse and watery for a few days. Vomiting occurs occasionally. Morbidity is high but mortality is low or absent. Moderate severity is observed in naïve sows and gilts, especially in those that have farrowed recently and are heavily exposed to virus from piglets with TGE. The dams show anorexia, vomiting, diarrhea, depression and may cease to lactate. Recovery usually occurs within 5-10 days.

Lesions

Gross lesions in baby pigs include marked dehydration, distension of the small intestine with foamy, yellow, odoriferous fluid and scattered milk curds. The intestinal wall is very thin and nearly transparent. The stomach may be empty because of vomiting but sometimes is filled with curdled milk. Chyle seldom is present in mesenteric lymphatics since fat absorption is impaired. There often are yellow or gray urates on the renal papillae. Watery colonic contents, often with undigested milk curd, usually have an acid pH. Microscopic alterations include a marked villous atrophy, perhaps with squamous metaplasia of epithelium, and elongation of crypts in scattered areas of the jejunum and ileum.

Diagnosis

In acute outbreaks involving young piglets, a tentative diagnosis often can be made on the basis of the explosive nature of a diarrheal disease accompanied by frequent vomiting and high mortality. The outbreaks often involve all ages of swine but high mortality is confined to small piglets. Lesions, including villous atrophy, also are helpful in diagnosis but not specific. Atrophic villi sometimes can be seen with a hand lens or dissecting microscope.

A specific laboratory diagnosis often can be made using a fluorescent antibody technique applied to fresh sections or scrapings of the jejunum or by immunohistochemistry on formalin-fixed sections. Confirmation of diagnosis requires samples be taken from euthanized pigs in the early stage of the disease. Polymerase chain reaction (PCR), when available, can be performed on feces from acutely affected pigs. This test is particularly valuable in postweaning pigs where fewer viruses are present, lesions are less severe, and disease is further advanced before clinical diarrhea is evident. Virus isolation in tissue culture followed by identification is possible but rarely done. Diseases that must be differentiated include colibacillosis, rotaviral or *Strongyloides* infection, coccidiosis and, where the disease occurs, porcine epidemic diarrhea.

Control

Preventive measures for negative herds include maintaining a closed herd and implementing strict biosecurity practices. Necessary additions should be from herds that have no recent history of TGE. Additions should be serologically negative before and after a quarantine period of 30 days. The all in/all out system of production with cleaning and disinfection between farrowings is helpful.

An owner may wish to eradicate TGE and maintain a negative herd after infection has occurred. This can sometimes be accomplished by whole-herd exposure to virus and allowing no introductions into the herd for a 60-day period. Alternatively, depopulation during a hot month should be accompanied by thorough cleaning and disinfection. Then, after allowing the facilities to be free of swine for several weeks, restocking with serologically negative stock may be effective.

Attenuated and killed virus vaccines are available. Vaccines usually are used to stimulate immunity in the dams although some also can be given to neonatal piglets. Vaccines are usually administered to dams at intervals prior to farrowing. All the vaccines currently available are most effective when used to stimulate an anamnestic response in previously exposed swine but are generally unable to protect a naïve population in the face of an acute exposure.

In acute outbreaks, pregnant sows and gilts that are two or more weeks from farrowing can be induced to form their own antibodies to TGE to protect their litter by purposefully infecting them with feces or piglet intestinal homogenates from the farrowing house. Antibodies in their colostrum and milk will then provide protection for the most critical time for their piglets. When possible, dams less than two weeks from farrowing should be farrowed separately in isolation.

Endemic TGE may follow an acute outbreak, particularly in larger herds where the whole herd is not simultaneously infected. The virus continues to infect susceptible animals (herd introductions and neonates), persists, and is often is difficult to prevent or eradicate. This form often occurs on premises where there are frequent farrowings or additions. On those premises it may be better to ensure exposure of all swine, especially breeding stock and replacements. Protocols exist for control and/or eradication of TGE in these endemic situations. Basically, all breeding swine should be exposed until they have shown signs of TGE. This can be done by feedback of minced intestine or contents from infected piglets on the premise. Those that do not show signs may have to be individually dosed orally. Vaccination can be an aid in sustaining immunity. All measures are more likely to succeed if a strict all in/all out system is practiced with thorough cleaning and disinfection of facilities between batches of pigs.

Piglets less than three weeks old with TGE seldom respond to treatment. Interventions include weaning, oral electrolytes, and a warm environment. Older swine usually recover spontaneously. Piglets at least one month old before onset usually recover if provided with a nutritious starter feed, warm housing and good care. Antibiotics added to feed or water might be of value in preventing secondary bacterial infections.

Vesicular Stomatitis

Definition
A vesicular viral disease capable of infecting cattle, horses, swine, people and many kinds of wildlife.

Occurrence
Vesicular stomatitis (VS) is endemic in various regions of North, Central, and South America. Widespread epidemics usually occur about every 10 years. The virus is endemic in sections of the southeastern U.S. but has not spread to swine. Most outbreaks of VS affect horses and cattle, less often swine. Infection also occurs in deer, bobcats, raccoons, feral swine and rodents.

Historical information
Vesicular stomatitis was first recognized in horses during the Civil War. In 1943, infection occurred in swine stemming from the use of VS-contaminated hog cholera serum. The endemic nature of VS in limited geographic areas and its epidemic nature in other areas remain unexplained by epidemiologists. The close resemblance of VS to foot-and-mouth disease and other exotic vesicular diseases continues to compel interest in the disease by animal health officials.

Etiology
Vesicular stomatitis is caused by a rhabdovirus. There are two serotypes of VS, Indiana and New Jersey (NJ). They do not cross immunize. Swine are susceptible to both serotypes. The Indiana serotype has three subtypes while the NJ serotype causes most major epidemics. VS virus is not considered to be highly contagious among domestic animals.

Epidemiology
The complete epidemiology of VS is not known. There may be unknown reservoirs and vectors of the virus, including insects. The disease remains endemic in certain river basins and coastal areas. In temperate zones, the appearance of VS usually coincides with the appearance of warm weather and ceases with the first frosts. This suggests virus is transmitted by insects, especially to horses and cattle, which frequently are infected while on pasture. Insect transmission is not essential; contact transmission has been observed. VS virus has been isolated from both biting and non-biting insects. Biting insects probably become infected by feeding on lesion areas although the viremic period is short. Non-biting insects may transmit virus mechanically. VS virus persists in feral swine and may provide virus for vectors.

The NJ strain of VS virus has been isolated from sandflies (*Lutzomyia shannoni*) and trans-ovarial transmission of virus has been demonstrated in sandflies. Movement of animals incubating or carrying virus may play a role in epidemics that occur far from endemically infected areas. Fomites from outbreaks in other species often have played a role in spread of VS to swine.

Pathogenesis
Virus appears to require introduction into epithelium through insect bites or abrasions of the skin. However, transmission may occur through the respiratory tract. Lesions appear initially as small, blanched papules. Lesions first develop in cells of the stratum spinosum and vesicles form. Epithelial cells above the stratum basale separate in about 30% of the cases. Loss of fluid through the stratum corneum results in inspissation (thickening by dehydration) of many lesions. The devitalized epithelium over vesicles soon erodes to leave shallow craters that fill with serum and erythrocytes. Since the basal layer of epidermis usually remains intact, most lesions soon heal. Gross and microscopic lesions of the vesicular diseases of swine are similar to those of other species and their morphology is not an adequate basis for differential diagnosis.

Clinical signs and lesions
Clinical signs are similar in all the vesicular viral diseases of most domestic species but there are a few differences peculiar to species and in the location of most lesions. Infection with VS virus stimulates a sharp rise in temperature that usually regresses after onset.

In swine, vesicles on the feet are common. Lameness is often the first sign that is noticed. Vesicles that form and coalesce around the coronary band may lead to loss of hooves, foot deformity and persistent lameness. Vesicles frequently occur on the snout and may extend into the nares. If lesions develop on the lips or in the mouth, there may be excessive salivation, slobbering and chomping. The vulva and scrotum occasionally have lesions. In nursing sows, vesicles may occur on the teats. Vesicles often develop at points of abrasion.

Vesicles usually rupture within 24 hours and the overlying epithelium detaches to leave shallow erosions with reddened or hemorrhagic surfaces. Lesions usually heal within two weeks unless secondarily infected with bacteria.

Pregnant sows may abort as a consequence of fever but none of the vesicular viruses have been reported to affect fetuses. Overall incidence is variable and mortality is low.

Diagnosis
Because signs and lesions of the vesicular viral diseases are similar, a variety of laboratory techniques have been developed for differential diagnosis. In the United States, the Federal Animal Disease Diagnostic Laboratory (FADDL) at Plum Island, NY usually is used for diagnosis. If signs or lesions consistent with VS are observed, state animal disease control offices should be contacted and will help make necessary arrangements for sample testing.

Epithelial and vesicular fluid samples can be used for complement fixation or enzyme-linked immunosorbent assay (ELISA) tests to identify viral antigen. Heparinized and clotted blood should be collected for virus isolation and identification, and for serologic testing respectively. A full set of tissues should be taken for histologic evaluation. Foot-and-mouth disease is of primary concern in differential diagnosis. If horses are affected, it is useful to know that horses are susceptible to vesicular stomatitis but not other vesicular viral diseases.

Control

Many laws that assist in control of VS are measures applicable to the control of all exotic diseases of livestock. They apply to all major categories of domestic animals. They control the importation of animal-derived food products, semen, embryos and biologics. In order to reduce the likelihood of spread of any of the vesicular viruses through garbage feeding, there are regulations that specify how garbage must be cooked before feeding it to swine. Other regulations are designed to prevent the discharge of garbage in ports.

Vaccines have not been used to control VS in swine although killed vaccines may be approved for use in cattle during an epidemic. Segregation of swine away from cattle and horses is an important, practical method of preventing spread of VS to swine. Control of flies, mosquitoes and other insects may be of value.

Emergency measures for control of outbreaks of vesicular diseases in swine require quarantine, identification of the disease, and slaughter of all infected and exposed swine. This is followed by a thorough cleaning and disinfection of the premises. For more information, see the table, Vesiculating Viral Diseases, on page 163.

Section III

Parasitic Diseases

Coccidiosis

Definition

A disease characterized by diarrhea in suckling and recently weaned pigs. The disease is usually caused by *Isospora suis* but occasionally by other *Eimeria* spp.

Occurrence

"Neonatal" coccidiosis caused by *Isospora suis* usually occurs in confinement-raised, one to three week old, nursing piglets and is less frequent and severe in older recently weaned piglets. Coccidiosis occurs in all countries where confinement rearing and continuous farrowing are practiced.

Although several coccidia of the genus *Eimeria* commonly infect one to three month old swine, clinical disease rarely occurs. Disease only occurs when previously unexposed pigs are placed in highly contaminated environments including unsanitary nurseries or grow/finish facilities.

Historical information

Although *Isospora suis* infection was identified as a cause of enteritis in 1934, it was not identified as a serious problem for swine raisers until the mid-1970s. Coccidiosis assumed greater importance with the introduction of confinement-rearing, continuous farrowing in warm buildings, and use of farrowing crates. These innovations facilitated rapid completion of the life cycle of *I. suis* in high numbers. Coccidiosis has re-emerged as a common cause of neonatal diarrhea, even in modern well-managed farms.

Etiology

Isospora suis is the usual cause of coccidiosis in very young, confinement-raised pigs. Oocysts become infective in about 12 hours at temperatures of 68-97°F. This is within the range maintained in many confinement farrowing facilities. After ingestion of sporulated oocysts, patency in neonatal pigs can occur in as little as five days.

Isospora suis goes through the usual stages of sporogeny, excystation, and endogenous development with multiplication in intestinal epithelium as is reported in other species. Development usually occurs in epithelium of the small intestine, especially in the jejunum and ileum, less often in the duodenum, cecum and colon. Development usually occurs in the cells on distal portions of intestinal villi; in severe infections it may occur in cryptal epithelium. Fully sporulated oocysts of *I. suis* have two sporocysts; each of these has four sporozoites. *Eimeria* spp. are quite similar but have a longer (18 day) life cycle and a higher affinity for the large intestine and distal small intestine.

Epidemiology

Coccidia are initially introduced into farrowing facilities by carrier sows. Oocysts produced by dams or more likely, their parasitized piglets, survive in farrowing rooms and crates and become a major source of infection for subsequent litters. Once infected, piglets magnify the numbers of oocysts and heavily contaminate the environment. As a result of this buildup of oocysts, piglets are able to ingest high numbers of oocysts, a requisite for producing clinical disease. Inadequate sanitary practices between farrowing groups undoubtedly facilitate this buildup.

In a warm, moist environment, oocysts in feces-contaminated farrowing rooms and crates soon become infective. They are ingested when piglets first nurse or when they ingest feed, water or feces in the farrowing crate. The sporozoites within oocysts mature and are released to penetrate enterocytes. Many enterocytes are destroyed by the developing coccidia. Released oocysts are passed in the feces.

Pathogenesis

The development of coccidia in enterocytes results in desquamation of enterocytes, especially those on the distal tips of villi. The severity of lesions is related to the number of oocysts ingested. Bacteria in the intestine, including *Clostridium*, may contribute to overall severity of the lesions. When many coccidia are ingested, lesions are severe. In serious infections, the erosion of villous epithelium results in loss of fluid and failure of surviving epithelium to absorb nutrients and fluids. This leads to diarrhea, dehydration, and loss of electrolytes, perhaps death.

Since regeneration of villous epithelium occurs more slowly in neonates, they are more severely affected. If piglets ingest only small numbers of oocysts, they survive and are immune unless stressful environmental or secondary infections intervene.

Clinical signs

Signs can occur as early as five days after birth but are more commonly seen in piglets from one to three weeks old. Signs include yellow to clear, pasty to watery diarrhea, dehydration, rough hair coat and failure to gain weight. The clinical disease within a litter can appear in two waves; the first wave (four to six days) representing infection and subsequent contamination of the farrowing crate environment by a few affected pigs, the second wave appearing four to eight days later after the rest of the litter becomes infected. Piglets usually continue to nurse but may vomit milk. Morbidity is high but mortality is variable, often moderate. Producers often report neonatal diarrhea that resembles colibacillosis but that fails to respond to antibiotic therapy. Fecal blood is not a feature of porcine coccidiosis.

Lesions

Lesions are usually restricted to the intestinal tract, especially the lower jejunum and ileum. Lesions vary in severity, depending on the number of oocysts ingested. In mild infections, the intestine tends to be turgid. Mild fibrinous enteritis may be visible in short segments of the lower small intestine. In severe infections, there may be extensive fibrinonecrotic enteritis. Occasionally the duodenum, cecum or colon are affected.

Microscopically, there is necrosis and, later, atrophy and fusion of some mucosal villi, hyperplasia of cryptal epithelium and elongation of mucosal crypts. Shortened villi may be covered by cuboidal or flattened epithelial cells. Various stages of *Isospora suis* are apparent in parasitized cells. If adequate time has elapsed since initial infection, there may be oocysts in the feces.

Diagnosis

Diagnosis can be made most reliably by identifying the coccidia in histologic sections. The presence of paired type-1 merozoites are considered diagnostic for *I. suis*. Several areas of infected mucosa should be examined in order to maximize sensitivity of the histological examination as distribution of microscopic lesions and merozoites is unpredictable.

Diagnosis by fecal examinations may be possible but is thought to be less sensitive than examination of affected small intestinal tissue. It is best attempted on piglets that have been sick two to three days so that oocysts have had time to develop. Feces collected at earlier or later stages of the disease may contain few or no oocysts. In fecal samples, either "hazy bodies" between the oocyst wall and the sporont, or oocysts in the 2-cell stage, are diagnostic for *I. suis*.

Coccidiosis can occur concurrently with other diseases so it may be necessary to eliminate them as additional causes of the diarrhea. These include rotaviral infection, colibacillosis, transmissible gastroenteritis, parasitism by *Strongyloides ransomi*, and infection with *Clostridium perfringens* type A or C.

Control

A vigorous, effective sanitation program, along with careful cleaning and disinfection of farrowing crates between farrowings is essential. Strong bleach or ammonium compounds can be used for disinfection after thorough cleaning of the crates. Between farrowings, steam cleaning of the entire farrowing facility may be necessary. Sealing all surfaces with paint or a water seal may be preferable to break the cycle of infection. Wooden and concrete surfaces are particularly difficult to clean effectively on affected farms. Installation of perforated metal or plastic flooring in the crates will be beneficial in the control of coccidiosis and other neonatal enteric diseases.

On farms known to be affected by coccidiosis, routine treatment of all piglets with toltrazuril early-on will minimize the incidence and severity of coccidiosis. There is no proven, widely accepted anticoccidial or drug for use in dams that is effective at controlling the disease in neonates.

Most cases of coccidiosis associated with *Eimeria* spp. are the result of the introduction of naïve pigs into a heavily contaminated environment. Control is based on minimizing the dose of oocysts ingested. Scrupulous sanitation between groups of pigs is usually sufficient to prevent disease.

Kidney Worm Infection

Definition
Infection of swine with the nematode worm *Stephanurus dentatus.*

Occurrence
Stephanurus dentatus infection occurs only in swine. All age groups, including fetuses, are susceptible. Pigs raised in tropical or subtropical areas on moist, shaded pastures are most often infected. In the United States, endemically affected areas include the area south of a line from the Carolinas westward to southern Missouri. However, the disease has occurred in feral and domestic swine in Canada and in other northern locations where southeastern pigs have been transported.

Historical information
Stephanurus dentatus infections once were common in several southern and southeastern states. However, good control of the parasite was realized once its life cycle was determined. A shift to raising a larger numbers of pigs in the Midwestern US, an area less favorable for *S. dentatus*, helped reduced incidence of infection. Indoor housing, confinement rearing and more effective parasiticides have further improved control.

Etiology
Adult kidney worms are 20-45 mm long and about 2 mm in diameter. They have a black and white mottling related to internal organs and their contents. Their life cycle is lengthy. Patency seldom is reached in less than 9-12 months and is usually only achieved in swine that reach breeding age. The mature parasites produce ova for at least three years.

The ova are thin walled, morulated, and measure 120 by 70 μm. Ova are passed in the host's urine. In a warm, moist, shaded environment, ova hatch in one to two days and larvae are infective in three to five days. Under favorable conditions, the larvae can survive for several months.

Epidemiology
Invasion by larvae can occur prenatally across the placenta, by skin penetration, ingestion in feed or, perhaps, by ingestion of earthworms. Ingestion probably is the most common route of infection.

Larvae go through five developmental stages (L1-L5) to reach maturity. Ingested L3 larvae migrate from the small or large intestine to various sites. Many travel via mesenteric lymphatics or by portal venous blood to the liver where they migrate extensively for two to four months. The larvae then penetrate the liver capsule, cross the peritoneal cavity and encyst in their definitive site: the perirenal fat or near ureters. Here they establish fistulous connections with the renal pelvis or ureters. When mature, they discharge their ova into the urine. Occasionally the parasites can be found within the kidney.

When infection by the L3 occurs transcutaneously, larvae first migrate to the lungs, then ascend the trachea to the pharynx, and finally are swallowed to reach the intestine. They then follow the same route followed by ingested larvae.

Development to patency usually takes at least 9-12 months after ingestion of larvae. Prenatal infections can result in patency in less than five months but this route of infection seems only to occur infrequently. Most swine are marketed before patency can occur.

Pathogenesis
Severe damage is caused by the migrating larvae. During migration through the portal vein, they often produce a severe phlebitis. Prolonged migration in the liver, prior to patency of the parasite, can cause severe interstitial hepatitis with extensive fibrosis. In slaughter age swine, hepatic fibrosis and abscessation can be extensive and lead to liver condemnation. Because larvae migrate widely, lesions are produced at many different sites.

Clinical signs
An unthrifty appearance, slow growth, poor feed conversion and occasional deaths in the herd are common signs. Other signs are usually seen only sporadically and reflect localization of larvae in aberrant sites. Posterior ataxia or paralysis occurs occasionally in pigs when larvae migrate in or along the spinal cord.

Lesions
Lesions depend somewhat on the stage of parasitism observed. Often the most obvious lesion is a gray to white, cirrhotic liver which may contain small abscesses. Lesions usually are more severe than those caused by the larvae of *Ascaris suum*. Additional lesions may include swelling of mesenteric lymph nodes, phlebitis in the portal vein with occasional thrombi, and small abscesses in the pancreas or lung. Other less common lesions include peritonitis (sometimes with intussusception of the intestine), pleuritis, and localized abscesses or abscess-like lesions in the spleen, lumbar muscles, retroperitoneum or spinal cord. Adult worms are most often found in or near the kidney, in walls of the ureters, or in the perirenal fat.

Diagnosis
Diagnosis is usually made at necropsy by observation of the abscesses and parasites at sites of localization. The extensively-scarred, enlarged liver seen with severe infestations is rather unique in swine and may suggest the diagnosis, especially in areas where the parasite is endemic. Diagnosis can be made in the live animal or at necropsy by identifying ova in the urine. The first urine passed in the morning often contains many ova.

Control
Control is possible through a breeding program that utilizes only gilts and young boars. These are slaughtered after producing one

litter. This usually precludes their living long enough for ova of *S. dentatus* to be passed in their urine. Eradication has been achieved on some production sites by this and management changes that preclude swine coming into contact with the parasite on pasture. Placing feeding and watering equipment on concrete in a sunny, well-drained location is a simple management practice that has value. Confinement housing usually eliminates losses from kidney worms.

Treating sows a few weeks prior to farrowing will usually prevent transplacental transmission of the parasite to fetuses. For treatment, see the table, Anthelmintics and Parasiticides, on page 147.

Louse Infestation (Pediculosis)

Definition
Infestation with the louse *Haematopinus suis.*

Occurrence
Infestation is common where husbandry and management are poor. The lice live only on swine although they may temporarily infest people handling swine. All age groups of swine are susceptible to infestation. Infestation is more severe in winter although it persists throughout the year. Presumably, the parasitism is worldwide wherever swine are raised.

Historical information
Prior to the development of good parasiticides, pediculosis in swine was very common. It was a common practice to use waste crankcase oil or diesel fuel as a topical spray on swine to reduce the number of lice. In at least a few instances, the practice resulted in terrible accidents when a match or cigarette was carelessly dropped where swine had been crowded together and soaked with these flammable liquids.

The relatively recent development of many effective parasiticides has made it possible for a producer to completely eradicate lice.

Products that control both internal and external parasites, including lice, have made control of lice more convenient.

Etiology
Haematopinus suis is one of the largest species of lice, up to 6 mm long. *Haematopinus suis* is a sucking louse and obtains blood meals from the host through its penetrating mouth parts. The louse spends its entire life on the host. It can survive off the host for only a few days. The female louse lives about 23-30 days, lays three to four eggs ("nits") per day and attaches them to hair shafts near their base. Eggs are 1-2 mm long and light cream to gray in color. They hatch in 12-20 days.

Epidemiology
Hog lice, like most lice, are host specific. They usually spread among swine when the pigs are in close contact, as when they crowd together for warmth, shade or comfort. Also, lice can spread to pigs moved into quarters recently vacated by lousy animals. Infested animals added to a clean herd often introduce lice.

Lice living on a pig have certain preferred sites because they prefer to feed on thin-skinned areas. Favorite sites include the neck, jowl, flank, the inner side of the legs and ears. In the ears, they often reside in "nests." Similar nests often are found on the abdomen, sometimes within the circles of pityriasis rosea lesions. Location within the ear offers lice protection from parasiticides because it is difficult to thoroughly wet the inner surface.

Pathogenesis
Lice annoy swine when they pierce the skin to take a blood meal. Dermatitis develops and leads to rubbing, scratching and some loss of hair. Loss of blood is not severe in most pigs but can lead to severe anemia in nursing pigs and may make them more susceptible to other diseases. Parasitized pigs are restless. They may lose weight and utilize feed less efficiently.

Lice are known vectors of agents that cause swine pox, African swine fever and eperythrozoonosis. It seems likely that other infectious agents may be transmitted as well.

Clinical signs
Persistent rubbing and scratching, patchy alopecia and pallor are signs of pediculosis. Because similar signs are seen with sarcoptic mange, it must be differentiated. Pediculosis and sarcoptic mange often occur concurrently. Hog lots and facilities with many rubbing sites also suggest that lice or mange are present.

Diagnosis
Lesions include a rough, dull hair coat, often with patchy alopecia. A thorough examination reveals the lice and ova attached to the hair. Examination of the inner aspect of the ears often reveals the lice and it also is a good place to look for sarcoptic mange lesions.

It is a good practice to occasionally pick up a few small and growing pigs, turn them over and examine their undersides. Lice, as well as lesions of several other diseases, often are readily apparent on the posterior abdomen or on the inside surface of the legs.

At slaughter and removal of hair, the punctate cutaneous lesions caused by feeding lice are visible, especially in white skinned hogs.

Control
Animals being introduced into a herd should always be treated with a parasiticide, preferably at least twice at two-week intervals, before being added to a herd. Many effective parasiticides are now available. A repeated treatment kills lice that emerge from eggs 12-20 days after an initial treatment.

Several parasiticides control external parasites other than lice (flies, mites and ticks). Injectable avermectins have been very effective in controlling both lice and mange and programs have been devised for eradicating both. See the table, Anthelmintics and Parasiticides, on page 147. Directions for use should be followed carefully. Some parasiticides require withholding periods prior to marketing.

Lungworm Infection (Metastrongylosis)

Definition
Infection with any one or more of three species of metastrongyle nematodes.

Occurrence
Swine can be infected by any of three different species of metastrongyles. All ages of swine are susceptible but heavy infections occur mostly in young pigs over six weeks of age. Infection is common in areas where pigs are raised outdoors with access to soil. Lungworms likely occur in all countries where swine and the intermediate host, the earthworm, is present.

Historical information
Lungworm infection historically was a major problem in US swine production. With the development of confinement housing and subsequent lack of access to soil (and earthworms), lungworm infection has decreased in prevalence. However, where pigs are raised in the outdoors, lungworm infection still can be a serious problem. Parasiticides effective in controlling lungworms, as well as many other parasites, have improved control. At one time, lungworms were erroneously believed to be important in the transmission of influenza virus to swine.

Etiology
Lungworms that infect swine include *Metastrongylus elongatus* (*apri*), *M. pudendotectus* and *M. salmi. Metastrongylus elongatus* infections are the most common but infection with more than one species can occur. Lungworms usually have an indirect life cycle through earthworms, but a direct cycle has been reported. Adult lungworms vary in length from 14-66 mm. They are white, threadlike and easily visible at necropsy. Lungworm ova are larvated, thick shelled, about 40 by 50 μm in size, and are passed in feces.

Epidemiology
First stage lungworm larvae hatch from eggs in swine feces and survive in feces or moist soil for long periods of time. In some areas the first stage larvae can survive over winter. After being ingested by earthworms, larvae are able to develop to the third infective stage in about 10 days. They then remain quiescent in the earthworm for up to 18 months. Thousands of larvae can accumulate in a single earthworm, apparently without harm to the earthworm.

Pigs on pasture root for earthworms, especially if the soil is soft and moist. Pigs ingest the parasitized earthworms and are infected by the larvae within them. The lungworm larvae penetrate the intestinal mucosa, migrate through lymphatics and venous blood and reach the lungs. There they localize, grow to maturity and produce larvated ova about 25 days after ingestion. Infection becomes patent in about four weeks. The larvated ova are coughed into the pharynx where they are swallowed and passed out through the feces.

Survival of lungworms depends largely on the survival of infective larvae in earthworms for long periods of time; also, on the ability of first stage larvae to survive for long periods in swine feces. Breeding and other older stock can remain infected for long periods and lungworm eggs in their feces continue contaminating the environment.

Pathogenesis
Third stage larvae penetrate the small intestine mucosa and pass in lymph and blood to the liver and lungs. Some larvae migrate in the liver and cause gray to white areas of scarring similar to those caused by ascarid migration. Larvae that reach the lungs break into alveoli where they mature, extending into terminal bronchioles. The parasites preferentially localize along the caudodorsal border of the diaphragmatic lobes. Their presence results in alveolitis and bronchiolitis leading to coughing. Exudate that forms around lungworms and their ova partially or completely obstructs airways resulting in alveolar emphysema and atelectasis. Secondary bronchopneumonia is a common sequela.

Clinical signs
Common clinical signs include chronic and sometimes paroxysmal coughing that eventually leads to generalized unthriftiness. If secondary pneumonia intervenes, there may be dyspnea and perhaps an abdominal type respiration ("thumping"). Signs are similar to those caused by ascarid migration in the lungs. The two parasitisms often occur concurrently where pastures are heavily contaminated by both ascarids and lungworms.

Lesions
Pigs with many lungworms are unthrifty, have a rough hair coat, and are small for their age. Pulmonary lesions often occur on the caudodorsal border of diaphragmatic lobes. When viewed from the dorsal aspect, those lesions often have a roughly triangular shape and appear as recessed darker areas of atelectasis or raised, lightly colored, emphysematous areas. Usually both types of lesions can be present in the same pig. If the distal border of the lobe is trimmed and lesion areas squeezed, adult worms can be expelled. The bronchial tree should always be opened as lesions along the border are not always present. When this is done, inflammatory exudate and lungworms may be found in terminal airways. Scattered 1- to 2-cm areas of gray-to-white scarring may be visible in the liver.

Diagnosis
Diagnosis is made most easily by postmortem examination of a few typical, affected pigs. Also, laboratory fecal exams usually will reveal the embryonated eggs of lungworms. Postmortem exams have the advantage of permitting examination for other parasites and diseases and often require less time.

Control

Prevention of heavy infection is possible by preventing access of pigs to soil that contains larvae or earthworms. Consequently, most confinement-raised pigs are free of lungworms.

Pigs raised outdoors often can avoid heavy infection if they are farrowed and raised on clean pastures. Pasture rotation is helpful but sometimes fails to prevent infection as lungworm larvae persist in earthworms for long periods of time. Using an effective anthelmintic on sows prior to farrowing and then moving them to clean pasture is helpful. There are several effective anthelmintics. See the table, Anthelmintics and Parasiticides, on page 147.

Mange (Sarcoptic Mange)

Definition
A parasitic disease of the skin caused by the sarcoptic mange mite and often characterized by marked pruritis and papules.

Occurrence
Sarcoptic mange occurs in all age groups but is inapparent in neonatal pigs until signs and lesions have had time to develop. It is likely the disease occurs in all countries where pigs are raised in large numbers. Sarcoptic mange is a common disease and represents the most important ectoparasitic disease of swine. Sarcoptic mange occurs in many other species but the mite *Sarcoptes scabiei* var *suis* is specific only for swine.

Historical information
Sarcoptic mange was first reported about 60 years ago. Little attention was paid to early reports; it was widely believed that scratching was natural and normal behavior for pigs. Also, economic loss caused by the disease was not widely appreciated. Intensification of production after World War II, along with greater attention to economics of production, focused attention on the avoidable losses caused by sarcoptic mange. Development of better and more convenient acaricides has greatly improved control.

Etiology
The mite *Sarcoptes scabiei* var *suis* causes most mange in swine. The mite is about 0.5 mm in length, gray to white, and just visible to the naked eye when on a black background. All stages of the mite (ova, larvae, nymphs, adults) develop in the epidermis. The life cycle is completed in about 10-15 days. Mites and ova survive away from the host for only short periods of time. Depending on temperature and humidity, this could be as short as one hour, or as long as 15 days.

Demodectic mange, caused by the mite *Demodex phylloides*, is unrelated to sarcoptic mange and relatively unimportant in swine. It is mentioned here because it occasionally causes dermatitis over the snout, inside the thighs and over the flanks. Occasionally it involves the whole body and leads to excessive trimming or condemnation at slaughter. Nodules caused by *D. phylloides* have been mistaken for swine pox.

Epidemiology
Mange in a herd usually develops after introduction of asymptomatic swine carriers. *Sarcoptes scabiei* var *suis* is rarely, if ever, transmitted from other species. If swine are moved immediately into quarters recently vacated by infested pigs, they are likely to become infested.

Spread is by direct body contact, often the result of pigs crowding together for warmth or shade. Mites from the dam often invade neonatal piglets within a few hours of birth.

Pathogenesis
Mites spread among pigs in close contact and invade the skin. They burrow through the epidermis where eggs are laid. The mites are a strong irritant to the skin and initiate severe scratching and rubbing. In about two to three weeks, an allergic hypersensitivity develops in many pigs causing them to rub and scratch even more vigorously, further traumatizing the skin.

Mites tend to first colonize the skin of the inner surface of the ear. From this site, they spread out over the body, tail and legs. Ear lesions first appear as small encrustations. These enlarge to form plaque-like lesions. Constant rubbing and scratching irritates the skin at many sites on the body and promotes hyperkeratosis and proliferation of connective tissue in the dermis. These lead to thickening, wrinkling and folding of the skin. Hyperkeratotic, gray to white patches often form on the irritated skin. Reddened macules and papules that develop on the skin of young growing pigs are thought to be related to hypersensitivity.

Clinical signs
Frequent rubbing and scratching are the usual signs. These signs often are more marked when the skin is first warmed by the sun, presumably the result of increased activity of mites. Signs of rubbing are often apparent on equipment or facilities which have been polished by rubbing pigs. Decreased rate of growth, inefficient use of feed and low sow productivity follow. Although morbidity is high, mortality from mange alone is unusual.

Lesions
Young pigs that have developed hypersensitivity to mange have reddened macules or papules, especially over the rump, flanks and abdomen. Chronic mange often affects relatively few older animals in the herd and is less pruritic. Lesions vary in extent and advanced cases can involve the skin over much of the body. The posterior aspect of the legs is often affected as those areas are easily scratched. In some cases, lesions may be mostly confined to the inner surface of the ears where hyperkeratotic areas often develop a brownish to red discoloration.

Diagnosis
Signs and lesions are suggestive of mange. Marked pruritis often helps differentiate mange from other diseases of the skin. Diagnosis can be confirmed by identifying the mites in skin scrapings or in exudate from the external auditory canal. Scrapings from the inner surface of the ear usually reveal more mites than do other sites. Scrapings are usually wetted with 10% potassium hydroxide, cover-slipped, and examined under a microscope using a low power objective. Another simple technique is to place the scraping on a piece of black paper for a few minutes. Then carefully blow off the superficial debris and examine the site on the paper for the small, light colored mites. Diseases that must be differentiated

from mange include parakeratosis, dermatomycosis, exudative epidermitis ("greasy pig disease"), pityriasis rosea, and photosensitization or sunburn.

Inspection of carcasses at slaughter may be useful, both in diagnosis and in evaluating the efficacy of a mange control program. An enzyme-linked immunosorbent assay (ELISA) test for serologic diagnosis of mange has been developed but is not widely available.

Control

Control programs should focus first on the breeding herd which, if infected, inevitably transmits mites to the piglets. These programs usually involve treatment of dams with external acaracide sprays or with an injectable avermectin a few days prior to entering the farrowing facility. Many farms using this control strategy find it necessary to also treat growing pigs at eight to ten weeks of age.

Eradication of mange is achievable in most production settings. Initiating an eradication program usually starts with culling of all severely infested breeding stock. Immediately following this, two consecutive doses of an injectable avermectin, 14 days apart, are administered to every pig on the farm (adults, neonates, and growing pigs). Removal of bedding material, if present, as well as application of an effective pesticide to environmental surfaces is often recommended at the same time injections are given. While eradication can be an expensive task in the short term, it is reliably efficacious and requires only standard biosecurity procedures to keep the mite from returning to the farm.

The avermectin class of parasiticides controls many external and internal parasites. One should carefully follow the directions that come with any product as some require a lengthy withholding period following their use. See the table, Anthelmintics and Parasiticides, on page 147.

Mycoplasma suis (Eperythrozoonosis)

Definition
A sporadic disease, usually observed in young, growing pigs, characterized by listlessness, fever, anorexia, hemolytic anemia and, in severe cases, by icterus.

Occurrence
Mycoplasma suis infection can occur in all age groups of swine but seldom is clinically apparent except in young, growing pigs. Serologic evidence indicates prevalence of less than 15% among swine with only a small number of outbreaks recognized. It often is associated with stress and can recur in stressed animals.

Outbreaks occur more often in the summer and often are concurrent with other infectious diseases, parasitisms or management problems. *M. suis* is likely to be species specific although the question has not been extensively researched. The geographic distribution of the disease is unknown. Relatively few countries have reported it.

Historical information
Icteroanemia in growing swine was described in the United States in 1943. At least four publications on *M. suis* infection were published in the 1950s. Recognition that there are many carriers came after development of an indirect hemagglutination test in 1975. *Mycoplasma suis* was thought to reside in the cell membrane but a report in 2009 indicated that *M. suis* can trasmigrate to the interior of the red blood cells. Although *M. suis* rarely causes spectacular death losses, it is recognized as an occasional cause of anemia or icterus in young pigs.

Etiology
The disease is caused by *M. suis* (previously *Eperythrozoonosis suis* and for a short time proposed to be renamed as *Mycoplasma haemosuis*), an obligate, intracellular bacteria. The organism is usually from 0.8 to 1.0 μm in diameter but may be larger during the acute stage of infection. It is predominantly coccoid-shaped but may appear rod or ring-shaped when viewed on an erythrocyte's cell membrane.

Epidemiology
There likely are numerous carriers in the swine population. Presumably, most of these are recovered animals that had *M. suis* infection in a subclinical form. In utero transmission has been demonstrated experimentally. The disease has been reported to occur in an acute form in sows immediately prepartum with piglets from sows also affected.

Since the disease occurs more frequently in the summer, it is suspected that mosquitoes and biting flies, as well as the hog louse (*Haematopinus suis*), play a role in transmission. The use of contaminated surgical instruments (including castration knives) and needles used repeatedly during vaccination are believed to transmit the organism. Ongoing infectious and parasitic diseases are believed to play an important role in precipitating outbreaks.

Pathogenesis
Much of the information on pathogenesis is based on study of experimental infection in splenectomized pigs. In these pigs, the clinical and pathologic aspects closely resemble natural infections. Once *M. suis* is introduced into the blood, a febrile response occurs in about 7-8 days. During the acute phase of the disease, *M. suis* organisms are numerous on the erythrocytes. Many infected pigs become hypoglycemic and some have convulsions, develop coma and die. A hemolytic anemia develops gradually, often requiring a week after onset before it is clinically apparent. Hemoglobinuria does not occur because hemolysis is extravascular. The number of platelets, the packed cell volume and hemoglobin values decrease. Under field conditions many affected animals recover but remain carriers.

Clinical signs
In young, growing pigs, prominent signs include anorexia, listlessness, marked weakness, pale mucous membranes and, perhaps, icterus. Temperatures are raised initially but often are subnormal by the time the pigs are examined. In chronic cases there often is marked icterus and deaths may occur. Signs in breeding stock are similar but are less obvious and often go unnoticed.

In breeding herds, *M. suis* infection has been associated serologically with various reproductive problems in breeding herds. However, proof that these were caused by the disease is lacking.

Lesions
At necropsy of young pigs, lesions depend somewhat on the duration of illness. Early cases exhibit pallor, watery pale blood, and perhaps modest enlargement of the spleen. In cold climates there may be necrosis of extremities. Hog lice, or their ova, often are present.

In older pigs the same lesions are apparent at necropsy but splenic enlargement is more noticeable. There often is icterus (more obvious internally) and it may be marked. The bone marrow is red, suggestive of hyperplasia. The liver often has a brownish cast from hemosiderosis. There often are suffusions in the abdomen, thorax and pericardial sac. Lymph nodes are edematous and swollen. The heart often is thin-walled and flabby. Careful examination often reveals lesions of concurrent diseases or parasitisms.

Diagnosis
M. suis is an unlikely cause of major disease. The history, signs and gross lesions often are of value in diagnosis. Confirmation is made by demonstrating the organisms in blood smears stained with Wright-Giemsa or Diff-Quick stains. The organisms are usually found on the surface of erythrocytes and/or in the plasma. Infection with M. *suis* must be differentiated from other causes of anemia. A careful search for concurrent diseases should be made. Differential diagnoses include systemic salmonellosis, porcine circovirus associated disease (PCVAD), mycotoxicosis, hepatotoxi-

cosis, iron deficiency anemia, or autoimmune hemolytic anemia.

Blood saved for smears to be examined by fluorescent microscopy should be collected in anticoagulant (heparin or acid citrate dextrose). One mL can be mixed with an equal part of 10% formalin. Smears made from this preparation can be stained with acridine orange. Blood collected during the early, acute stage of the disease has many more *M. suis* organisms than blood from chronic cases. Serologic tests (indirect hemagglutination, IHA; or enzyme-linked immunosorbent assay, ELISA) and polymerase chain reaction (PCR) may be available to confirm *M. suis* as a herd problem, although these tests have limited availability. Infected pigs less than three months old seldom react on IHA.

Control

Tetracyclines and organic arsenicals have been used with success for prevention and treatment of *M. suis* infections. Intracellular organisms may not be responsive to tetracycline treatments. Organic arsenicals should be used cautiously and directions followed carefully. They should not be given initially to thirsty pigs or poisoning may result. Their use has been associated with deafness in breeding animals.

Affected pigs can be treated individually with injectable oxytetracycline.

The indirect hemagglutination test can been used as a screening test prior to purchase of breeding stock or to identify herd infection. Neither IHA, ELISA nor PCR tests are widely available.

There are no vaccines for the prevention of *M. suis*.

Nodular Worm Infection (Oesophagostomiasis)

Definition

Infection of swine with parasites of the genus *Oesophagostomum.*

Occurrence

Nodular worms are distributed worldwide and, at least historically, frequently caused disease in swine, sheep and cattle. The species that occur in sheep and cattle do not pose a threat to swine. Roundworms, whipworms, and nodular worms are the most common internal parasites found in swine. Nodular worm parasitism usually only occurs in pigs raised in open lots or pasture but can rarely occur in confinement-raised pigs, including those without exposure to soil. The infection occurs in all age groups but pigs over three months old may be more susceptible.

Historical information

At one time, natural sausage casings were made from swine intestines from which the mucosa had been removed. Nodules from nodular worms made the preparation of the casings a difficult or impossible task. Natural sausage casings from swine are seldom used anymore.

Etiology

There are 5 species of *Oesophagostomum. Oesophagostomum dentatum* and *Oesophagostomum quadrispinulatum* are the two species that cause most disease in swine in the United States. Three other species are largely restricted to southeastern states.

Adult *Oesophagostomum* are 1-2 cm long, have slightly curved bodies and are white to gray. Their life cycle is direct although there are 2 non-parasitic stages that precede the parasitic stages. Ova are morulated and thin-shelled, about 70 by 40 µm. Under favorable conditions, non-parasitic stage larvae can persist on pastures for up to a year. Ingested L3 larvae penetrate the mucosa of the cecum and colon, molt to L4 larvae and return to the intestinal lumen in 6-20 days. Patency is reached as early as three weeks after ingestion; large numbers of ova are then passed in the feces.

Epidemiology

Survival of the parasite is facilitated by the ability of non-parasitic stages of larvae to survive on pastures and by the large number of ova laid. During the periparturient period, the number of ova passed in the feces increases substantially. This increase continues throughout the lactation period and almost ensures that some of the piglets will be infected.

Although ingestion of L3 larvae from contaminated pastures is the usual route of transmission between pigs; introduction of infected animals is the primary mode of between-herd transmission.

Pathogenesis

Ingested third stage larvae (L3) penetrate the mucosa of the cecum and colon and cause petechial hemorrhages and mucosal irritation. Most of the larvae penetrate to the base of the mucosa, encyst there and destroy part of the adjacent muscularis mucosae. The parasites then reside in both the mucosa and submucosa. Some larvae penetrate much more deeply, even to the serosa where adhesions may develop.

Larvae in the wall of the intestine stimulate a marked inflammatory reaction and an effort is made by the host to wall them off. Repeated invasions probably result in hypersensitivity that contributes to the reaction. Inflammatory edema with thickening of the mucosa and thrombosis of lymphatics often results. Although many of the parasites molt and return to the surface of the mucosa, some parasites are walled off and eventually destroyed. The fibrotic nodules formed around the parasites may persist for some time. Secondary infections of the nodules often occur.

Clinical signs

Most infections are asymptomatic. Others are concealed by signs of other parasitisms, especially ascariasis. Heavily infected animals may have diarrhea, decreased weight gain and poor feed efficiency. Deaths from nodular worm infection seldom occur.

Lesions

The intestinal wall of a heavily parasitized pig is thickened and edematous. In the cecum and colon, nodules up to 20 mm in diameter are scattered in the mucosa/submucosa and some may be apparent on the serosa. Nodules often contain necrotic debris. Mature parasites that successfully migrate back to the lumen are 1-2 cm long. The lesions are easily confused with dilated lymphoglandular complexes which are common in the colon of pigs with chronic bacterial enteritis.

Diagnosis

Diagnosis can be made on postmortem examination. Nodules in and on the large intestine and the presence of adult parasites in the lumen can be easily recognized. Lesions must be differentiated from abscessed lymphoglandular complexes.

Fecal exams can also be used for diagnosis. The eggs must be differentiated from grain mite eggs and from eggs of other Strongyloididae. Differentiation from *Hyostrongylus rubidus* may require larval culture.

Control

Nodular worm infection usually is controlled by the use of anthelmintics. Deworming sows prior to farrowing will reduce future exposure of the piglets. In confinement operations, frequent removal of feces and good sanitation also reduce exposure of dams and piglets. In outdoor operations, lots and pastures that are heavily contaminated should be avoided. Pasture rotation, with tillage of land when not pastured, is helpful. A large number of anthelmintics are available for control. See the table, Anthelmintics and Parasiticides, on page 147.

Roundworm Infection (Ascariasis)

Definition

Ascariasis is the infestation of swine by the roundworm, *Ascaris suum*, which can cause pneumonia, hepatitis, and ill thrift.

Occurrence

Ascariasis occurs worldwide in countries that raise significant numbers of swine. All ages are affected but ascariasis is more severe in young, growing pigs. It is the most prevalent and most economically important internal parasite of swine.

Migration of ascarid larvae occurs in several other animals, including man, but larvae usually do not develop to the adult stage in the intestine of these species. Migrating larvae occasionally infect lambs and calves and cause heavy losses from pulmonary lesions.

Historical information

The ascarid of man, *A. lumbricoides*, was once believed to be the same parasite as *A. suum*. However, *A. suum* is now recognized as a separate species. Effective control of ascarid infection came only after the life cycle was elucidated and interventions based on that knowledge were used to prevent infection.

Etiology

Mature ascarids are 15-40 cm long, thick bodied, round worms. A mature ascarid (prepatent period of seven to eight weeks) can lay almost two million eggs per day. Adults live in a pig for about six months before spontaneous expulsion begins but may survive a year or longer. Heavy infections can result in hundreds of ascarids in the intestine of a single pig.

Ascarid eggs are thick shelled, yellowish brown, almost spherical, 50-80 by 40-60 μm, and are coated with a sticky proteinaceous cover. The eggs are quite resistant to environmental degradation and disinfectants but can be destroyed by intensive steam cleaning or prolonged exposure to full sunlight.

Epidemiology

A. suum eggs are extremely hardy and can survive for as long as 15 years in the environment. They remain viable in swine effluent water for at least 14 months. The eggs can be transported by infested pigs, insects, fomites, blowing dust, pig manure, and effluent. Eggs are often disseminated through the feces of purchased swine, including breeding stock.

Ascarid eggs are ingested and hatch in the intestine. The larvae penetrate the mucosa, and pass through the bloodstream to the liver, lungs and other sites. They reach the liver two to four days after ingestion and are present in lungs within ten days. Once arriving in the lung, they break into alveolae, are coughed up the airways to the pharynx and are re-swallowed. The larvae reach the intestine 14-20 days after being initially ingested as eggs and become mature approximately two months later. Ascarids are prolific egg-layers with a prepatent period of approximately eight weeks, at which time eggs begin to be passed in feces. Eggs require two to four weeks in the environment for maturation before they become infective.

Once a location is infested, ascariasis persists in the pig population despite all measures used to eliminate it. The extremely high number of eggs that are produced, the resistance of eggs to environmental degradation, and the multiple means in which they can be disseminated contribute to their persistence on infected farms.

Low levels of ascarid exposure will stimulate a protective immunity. The most severe consequences of ascarid infection occur when immunologically naïve pigs are placed into contaminated sites. Farrowing and nursery facilities often have a low prevalence of ascarid egg contamination such that young pigs will have had little or no exposure to the parasite. Hence, these animals are at risk of severe disease when subsequently placed in contaminated finishing barns.

Pathogenesis

Ascarids cause local inflammation in the intestine and compete with the host for nutrients. This adversely affects growth of pigs, especially those on marginal or poorly balanced diets. With heavy infections, the most significant effect of the disease is a result of the migrating larvae causing lesions in the liver and lungs, including scarring of liver and interstitial pneumonia.

In the lungs, larvae break out of capillaries into alveoli. This results in small hemorrhages and an inflammatory reaction that interferes with the clearance mechanism of airways and favors secondary bacterial infections. Larvae rarely are carried to ectopic sites, e.g. the retina or brain, which may cause signs of impaired vision or central nervous system (CNS) lesions.

Ascarids are known to produce immunosuppressive substances that affect the duration and severity of other swine diseases and also may influence the response of swine to vaccines. Although difficult to quantify, there is evidence that ascariasis increases the severity of acute erysipelas and mycoplasmal pneumonia.

Clinical signs

Signs in young, growing pigs include unthriftiness, failure to gain weight, rough hair coat, pendulous abdomen, chronic paroxysmal coughing and occasionally, abdominal expiratory dyspnea ("thumping").

Severe, sometimes fatal, respiratory disease may result in 7-14 days after naïve pigs (feeder pigs or breeding stock previously unexposed) are placed in facilities heavily contaminated with ascarid eggs. Affected pigs are afebrile, "thump," are gaunt, and are often misdiagnosed as having bacterial or viral pneumonia. Other effects in heavily exposed gilts include delayed estrus, poor conception rate, pneumonia or death.

Lesions

By 5-14 days after ingestion of infective eggs, there are small hemorrhages on and throughout the lungs. Larvae and inflammatory exudate obstruct smaller airways (verminous pneumonia). Often, there is a secondary suppurative bronchopneumonia. The pneumonia may be accompanied by emphysema that interferes with collapse of the lungs. Scarring in the liver first appears by 7-14 days after exposure as scattered, gray to white "milk spots" (0.2-1 cm) visible under the liver capsule that later expand, coalesce and can eventually resolve. In heavy infections, diffuse fibrosis may affect the entire liver and lead to its condemnation at slaughter. Minor areas of scarring can be repaired in 30 to 60 days, making diagnostic reliability of detecting an absence of liver lesions at slaughter dubious.

Diagnosis

Diagnosis of chronic infestation (more than two months) can often be made by identifying eggs using fecal flotation examinations or by finding grossly visible ascarids in the small intestine. Since ascarids have some mobility, they sometimes can be found in the stomach or in the major bile and pancreatic ducts at necropsy. Obstruction of the bile duct sometimes leads to marked generalized icterus. Ascarids may not be present in animals recently "dewormed" but scarring in the liver or hemorrhages in the lung may still be apparent.

Diagnosis of acute infestations (less than two months) requires postmortem examination of a few typical pigs that have died or been sacrificed. Fecal flotations are not reliable during the first 6-8 weeks following infestation (prepatent period). Postmortem examination also permits the evaluation of concurrent diseases, including other sources of parasitism or causes of pneumonia. Diagnosis of early infestations is by observation of typical liver and lung lesions with confirmation by histopathology.

Control

A complete knowledge of the life cycle of ascarids and the infestation status of a herd or group of pigs is required to make timely and economical deworming decisions.

Prevention of ascariasis is far better than treatment but may be difficult to achieve on many production sites. Swine raised in confinement with a good ascariasis control program usually have few ascarids. Some of the measures that confinement operators implement include: deworming the sows during gestation (usually about a week before farrowing); washing the sows to remove parasite eggs prior to putting them in sanitized farrowing crates; early weaning of two to four week old pigs (before ascarid eggs have become infective); and using all in/all out production systems with thorough cleaning between groups.

Often, pigs produced in sanitary confinement systems are free of ascarid infection until placed in contaminated grow/finish facilities. These pigs then may develop severe pneumonia as they ingest numerous eggs from the environment. Feeding a continuous dewormer (pyrantel) for the first 30 days is a control option in this situation. Pigs in such conditions should be dewormed at no greater than eight-week intervals to prevent additional egg contamination of the site.

In operations that utilize pasture or open lot housing, deworming the sows before moving them to clean pasture is a good practice. Pasture rotation will greatly reduce the exposure of swine to worm eggs, especially if the land is tilled when not pastured. Deworming programs need to be designed to fit the situation on each production site.

Anthelmintics should be selected on the basis of the entire spectrum of nematode species present on the farm, including ascarids. A monitoring system should be established and followed. Sometimes the parasite problem changes as a consequence of introduction of other kinds of parasites, facility changes, or climatic changes which may influence the number and variety of parasites. See the table, Anthelmintics and Parasiticides, on page 147.

Thorny-headed Worm Infection

Definition
Infection by parasitic worm *Macracanthorhynchus hirudinaceus.*

Occurrence
This parasite occurs only in swine. Infection is usually seen in feeder or finishing pigs. These pigs are typically old enough to have had opportunity to root and forage, thus having access to the larvael stages of beetles. Infection is relatively common in pigs raised outdoors in southern states.

Historical information
The parasite was once believed to be a parasite only in southern states, but it is now found farther north into the lower Midwestern states.

Etiology
Macracanthorhynchus hirudinaceus has an elongated, sack-like body with no internal alimentary canal. There is a protrusible proboscis armed with about six rows of spiny hooks for attachment to the intestinal wall. The worms are 10-40 cm long, and up to 9 mm wide. They are transversely wrinkled, slightly curved, light pink and attenuated posteriorly. The brown ova are up to 110 by 65 µm and have a three-layered shell. The ova are resistant to environmental degradation.

Epidemiology
The eggs are passed and persist in swine feces. The eggs are ingested by beetles, their grubs or other arthropods that act as intermediate hosts. Swine then ingest these intermediate hosts. The eggs hatch in the intestinal tract of the pig and the worms attach there, usually in the ileum. The parasites develop by absorbing nutrients from the ingesta.

Pathogenesis
The worm's proboscis is inserted deeply into the wall of the intestine. It sometimes penetrates into the peritoneal cavity and introduces infection that leads to peritonitis. Intestinal bacteria usually infect the attachment site and an inflammatory nodule develops around it. The parasite occasionally moves to a new feeding site. The lesions cause hemorrhage, loss of blood proteins and localized intestinal infections. Animals with only a few parasites appear not to be seriously affected. Animals with many parasites tend to become unthrifty from loss of blood, the toxic effect of many localized lesions, and impaired nutrition.

Clinical signs
There are few or no signs with light infections. Pigs with heavy infections become unthrifty and have rough hair coats. Occasionally a parasitized pig dies as a consequence of intestinal perforation followed by peritonitis.

Lesions
Scattered inflamed nodules one to two cm in diameter are apparent through the serosa of the small intestine, usually the ileum. Attached worms often are large enough to be palpated through the unopened intestine. In the opened intestine, the sites that worms recently vacated appear as deep, infected ulcers. Old, healed sites appear as firm, fibrous nodules. The parasites are easily found and to the uninitiated, are spectacular in size, up to 40 cm long.

Diagnosis
Diagnosis usually is made at necropsy by finding and identifying the parasites. Alternatively, diagnosis can be made through laboratory fecal examinations

Control
Control is through avoidance of exposure to contaminated lots or pastures and to beetles, the usual intermediate hosts. Beetles should be eradicated around feed storage areas and other sites accessible to the swine. There is little data on treatment but levamisole has been recommended. See the table, Anthelmintics and Parasiticides, on page 147.

Threadworm Infection (Strongyloidosis)

Definition
Parasitism of swine by *Strongyloides ransomi*.

Occurrence
Infection with *S. ransomi* occurs only in swine. The parasite has a cosmopolitan distribution and is of importance in warmer countries or areas. It does not occur frequently in most areas of the United States. Although infection occurs in all age groups, including fetuses, pathogenicity usually is confined to nursing piglets.

Historical information
Most references to threadworm infection in swine are from the 1960s and 1970s. There are few recent publications. This suggests that current losses attributable to the parasite in the US are relatively minor. Environmental requirements of the parasite apparently restrict its spread.

Etiology
Only asexual females of *Strongyloides ransomi* are important in parasitism of swine. Free-living generations can produce progeny that are free living (heterogonic cycle) or progeny that are parasitic (homogonic cycle). Free-living generations can alternate with parasitic generations.

The asexual females are almost microscopic, about 3.3-4.5 mm long, and live in the mucosa of the anterior small intestine, usually the duodenum. The ova are thin shelled, larvated and are passed in the host's feces. Infective larvae hatch in one to two days. They require warmth and moisture for survival and are usually eliminated by desiccation, sunshine and good sanitary practices.

Epidemiology
Three mechanisms tend to assure survival of the parasite. These include the ability of *S. ransomi* to survive for some time in a non-parasitic form, four possible routes of transmission, and the ability to achieve patency in piglets in only a few days.

Parasitic larvae invade the host either by penetration of the skin (percutaneous), ingestion in feed (oral), ingestion in colostrum (transcolostral), or through direct invasion of developing fetuses (transplacental/perinatal). In all cases, the asexual female reaches the mucosa of the small intestine where many ova are produced and passed in feces of the host.

Larvae sequestered in muscle or in the mammary fat of sows are mobilized in the periparturient period and transmitted to piglets in colostrum. This is the most common route of transmission to neonatal piglets. Larvae in colostrum arrive at the intestinal mucosa without migration. Larvae also are transmitted directly to fetuses, presumably during the periparturient period.

Larvae that penetrate the skin enter the blood stream and are carried to the lungs. After breaking out into alveoli and tracheal migration to the pharynx, they are swallowed and reach the small intestine. Larvae taken into the mouth penetrate the mucous membranes of the oral cavity and, after a similar migration, reach the small intestine.

Pathogenesis
Adults that develop in the small intestine irritate the intestine, with the severity depending upon the number of parasites. The parasites cause a blunting and atrophy of intestinal villi. These alterations result in leakage of proteins into the gut and failure of the intestine to effectively absorb nutrients and fluids. The alterations lead to anemia, diarrhea, dehydration and emaciation. Migration of larvae through the lungs causes small hemorrhages as well as thickening and inflammation of alveolar septa that impair respiration.

Clinical signs
In mild infections there are few or no signs. In severe infections of neonatal piglets, there is anemia, diarrhea, dehydration, emaciation and deaths. Most mortality occurs in piglets less than two weeks old. Diarrhea, dehydration and unthriftiness can occur in pigs up to three months old.

Lesions
These are not readily apparent on gross examination. On microscopic examination of the small intestine, there is villous atrophy and blunting. Adult parasites can be seen in tunnels in the epithelium of glandular crypts of the mucosa. In the lung there is inflammation and thickening of alveolar walls, scattered hemorrhages, and perhaps migrating larvae. Neither hemorrhages nor larvae are numerous.

Diagnosis
Diarrhea in nursing pigs may suggest the possibility of infection with *S. ransomi*. However, all other common causes of diarrhea must be excluded first, especially infections with rotavirus, *Escherichia coli*, *Clostridium perfringens* and *C. difficile*, and coccidiosis. *Strongyloides ransomi* can often be identified in mucosal scrapings or histologic sections. The thin-shelled larvated ova can be identified by laboratory fecal examination but must be differentiated from larvated ova of lungworms (*Metastrongylus spp*).

Control
Avoidance of pastures with an environment favorable to the parasite will reduce exposure of sows and piglets. Indoor housing and confinement rearing, combined with maintenance of good sanitation, will reduce the likelihood of threadworm infection. Avermectins given to the sow a week or two prior to farrowing will control transmission of larvae to fetuses. For additional options, see the table, Anthelmintics and Parasiticides, on page 147.

Trichinellosis

Definition
Trichinella spiralis is a parasite that infects swine, other carnivorous animals, and people. The parasites are usually ingested through consumption of infected meat.

Occurrence
Most carnivorous, warm-blooded animals can become infected with the parasite. Infected animals of special importance in human trichinellosis include animals whose flesh is consumed raw or incompletely cooked (feral pigs, bears, several sea mammals, and horses). Species of particular importance, as sources of infection for swine, include previously infected pigs, rodents, and scavenged wildlife carcasses. Meat scraps from infected, slaughtered animals in uncooked garbage can remain infectious and may end up being a source of infection for commercial swine in some countries.

The incidence of infection in swine is low in countries that routinely inspect meat for *T. spiralis*. In the United States, food safety and eradication efforts have resulted in a prevalence so low that it is nearly undetectable with current diagnostic tests..

Historical information
Trichinellosis once caused outbreaks of severe illness in people but control measures were developed and adopted by many pork-producing countries. In some countries *T. spiralis* infection of swine is near eradication and this has suppressed outbreaks. In the United States, less stringent measures have greatly reduced trichinellosis in both pigs and people but the disease still occurs occasionally. In recent years, most of the US human cases are from eating game meat (especially bear meat) and not from pigs.

The FDA has approved irradiation of pork, beef and lamb. Irradiation kills trichinae as well as most bacteria that cause food poisoning. Research on *T. spiralis* and irradiation of pork products are driven by public health concern and a desire to expand foreign markets for pork. Swine production with trichinella-free certification is becoming a reality.

Etiology
The parasite is *Trichinella spiralis*. Four separately named strains of *Trichinella spiralis* have been named. They have minor anatomical differences and may simply represent different ecotypes of the same species.

Mature *T. spiralis* females are three to four mm long and are found in the duodenal and jejunal mucosa. A fertilized female produces 500-1000 larvae over a period of two to six weeks.

The parasite's life cycle begins with ingestion of infected muscle that contains encysted *T. spiralis* larvae. Trichinae within muscle fibers are liberated when cyst walls are exposed to gastric secretions after consumption. The larvae reach maturity in the small intestine in about four days. They mate and mature females penetrate into the mucosa and liberate larvae in lymphatics. Some larvae escape into the lumen of the gut and are eliminated in feces. Recently voided feces may be infectious but this is considered a minor mode of transmission.

Larvae in the lymphatics soon gain access to the systemic circulation. Many are destroyed by body defenses. Those that gain access to muscle fibers penetrate them, usually one per fiber. A larva within a fiber often induces a change in the fiber that causes it to enlarge and act as a nurse cell. In two to three months the larva reaches a length of over 100 µm and is enclosed in a cyst-like structure in the modified muscle cell. Here it can survive for up to 11 years.

Larvae have a predilection for certain striated muscles, generally those that normally are quite active, e.g. diaphragm, intercostal, lingual, laryngeal, masseter and ocular muscles. The larvae occasionally localize in cardiac muscle fibers. Once encysted, larvae must be ingested by another mammal for the cycle to be repeated.

Epidemiology
Survival of *T. spiralis* is promoted by the wide range of animals that serve as intermediate hosts, by the long survival of larvae in muscle fibers, and by the scavenging, cannibalistic nature of pigs.

In swine, transmission often occurs when pigs scavenge trichinella-infected carcasses of swine, rats or other animals. Transmission also occurs when uncooked garbage containing pork or other meat scraps that harbor *T. spiralis* are fed to pigs. Tail-biting of infected pigs and ingestion of larvae in feces are other possible sources of exposure.

Pathogenesis
Trichinella spiralis has a relatively low pathogenicity for swine but can cause severe clinical signs in people.

Clinical signs
Clinical signs seldom are observed in swine naturally infected with *T. spiralis*. Experimentally infected swine show signs of intense muscle pain and have decreased weight gains but most recover and weight gain improves. In infected miniature swine, hypergammaglobulinemia and eosinophilia have been reported.

Lesions
In swine, gross lesions are usually not visible unless there is white streaking from calcification of affected muscle fibers. On microscopic exam, the encysted parasites are easily observed. If there are degenerate or necrotic muscle fibers, an inflammatory reaction with many eosinophils may be present around them.

Diagnosis
The prevalence in the US swine population is low (0.007% in 2000) and usually no special effort is made to detect *T. spiralis* in slaughtered swine. In many countries, techniques used for

surveillance include trichinoscopic examination of muscle (often diaphragm muscle) likely to contain *T. spiralis* larvae. In this test, the muscle is homogenized and enzymatically digested in order to release the larvae from their cysts for efficient visualization by the technician. An enzyme-linked immunosorbent assay (ELISA) test and PCR are also available. *Trichinella*-free production certification in the US currently relies on an ELISA test.

Control

In the US, an educational program that places emphasis on thorough cooking of pork has been reasonably successful in minimizing the incidence of human infection. Also, there are regulations that govern the way ready-to-eat pork products must be processed to ensure destruction of *T. spiralis*. Irradiation of pork and other meats was legalized in 1988 and now is providing additional protection. A Pork Quality Assurance (PQA Plus) program, encourages good production practices that make *T. spiralis* infection in swine unlikely. It has been implemented by many producers and is required by some pork processors. In late 2008, the United States Department of Agriculture's Animal and Plant Health Inspection Service (USDA-APHIS) established a voluntary Trichinae Certification Program for US pork. Most recent reports of human trichinellosis in the US have been attributed to the consumption of undercooked wild game meat rather than commercial swine.

No effort should be made to treat animals suspected of having trichinellosis. They should be reported to state public health and animal health authorities.

Whipworm Infection (Trichuriasis)

Definition
Infestation of swine with whipworms, *Trichuris suis*.

Occurrence
Trichuris suis infections occur in domestic and feral swine; infection has also been reported in some primates, including man. Infection is relatively common in swine raised on pasture or in dirt lots. In the United States, whipworms were one of the three most prevalent internal parasites of swine, based on examination of several thousand fecal samples submitted to laboratories between 1988 and 1994.

All age groups are susceptible but most infestations occur in swine less than six months old. In adults, clinical signs can be induced when infection occurs in the face of severe stress. However, whipworms commonly infest adult pigs at a subclinical level and serve as a major source of infection for other swine. All major swine-producing countries have whipworm.

Historical information
Whipworm infections were common historically when more swine were raised outdoors on pasture or in previously used lots. In situations where that method of production is still practiced, whipworm infection is still common. Rearing swine in a confinement setting, without access to contaminated soil or feces from previous groups, has led to elimination of whipworms as a significant problem for most producers. In outdoor operations, newer anthelmintics have allowed for improved control over this once-troublesome parasite.

Etiology
Trichuris suis is the etiologic agent of whipworms in swine. Mature female whipworms are six to eight cm long, and males are about half that length. The life span of adults is four to five months. The anterior two-thirds of the parasite is quite thin and, when seen at necropsy, is buried in the mucosa of the intestine; the posterior one third is visibly thicker and usually seen protruding into the intestinal lumen. Worms are not visible grossly until at least three weeks post-infection.

Microscopically, ova are approximately 65 by 25 µm, yellow to brown in color, double operculated, and easily recognized. Ova passed in feces become infective in three to four weeks. The prepatent period is seven to eight weeks but clinical signs can be observed within one to two weeks of severe infestation. Ova production tends to be sporadic and there are times when there are few ova in the feces.

Epidemiology
Although adult worms have a relatively short life span and lay ova only sporadically, ova remain infective in most environments for up to six years. This long period of survival tends to perpetuate the species, even if pasture rotation is practiced. Adult swine tend to harbor low levels of infection resulting in a continual source of ova contamination in the environment.

Pathogenesis
After ingestion of larvated eggs, L3 larvae hatch and enter the mucosa of the anterior small intestine. The larvae reside there temporarily, return to the intestinal lumen for a period of time, then deeply reinvade the mucosa or submucosa of the cecum and colon. This penetration results in diffuse mucofibrinous to mucohemorrhagic typhlocolitis. Focal ulcerations may be complicated by secondary invasion of microorganisms that include salmonellae and the protozoan, *Balantidium coli*. Secondary infection often is an important part of the disease process.

The inflammatory reaction around the parasites results in edematous thickening of the wall of the gut and the formation of inflammatory nodules around some parasites. In heavy infections, a fibrinous pseudomembrane may form on the mucosa. Regional lymph nodes may be swollen as a consequence of drainage of toxic products.

Clinical signs
Clinical effects are directly related to severity of infestation and presence of concurrent diseases. Mild infestations are subclinical. Signs include anorexia, mucoid or mucohemorrhagic diarrhea, dehydration, and possibly death of severely affected animals. Signs are most apparent two to four weeks following exposure to contaminated facilities.

Lesions
During early stages (one to three weeks post-infestation) whipworms are not visible as they migrate within the mucosa. There is a mucoid to mucohemorrhagic typhlocolitis with excessive mucus, fibrin and blood on the mucosa. Lesions vary in extent from focal to diffuse and in acute stages, often resemble those of swine dysentery. The affected gut wall is thickened and edematous. Histopathology is required for diagnosis and will reveal the migrating larvae. Later, maturing whipworms become visible with careful gross examination. Worms often protrude from inflammatory nodules in the gut wall and purulent exudate may be visible around them. Gentle traction on parasites will free them from the gut wall, revealing the thin anterior end buried in the mucosa. Dilated lymphoglandular complexes should not be mistaken as lesions of either whipworms or nodular worms. Inflammation of the cecal and colonic walls can be quite extensive and severe even when only few adult worms are observed.

Diagnosis
Diagnosis is accomplished by necropsy of a typically affected pig. Mature parasites are easily found in the cecum or colon and can be identified by their size and whip-like form. Immature worms can cause severe lesions if numerous. They are much smaller than adults. For identification, they require careful observation, perhaps with the aid of flotation over a dark background or use of a magnifying lens. Extensive lesions of the immature worms in mucosal

migrations closely resemble and must be differentiated from those of swine dysentery, salmonellosis and proliferative enteritis, any of which may be concurrently present.

The presence of ova can be determined by laboratory fecal examinations by seven weeks after infestation but clinical signs and lesions will often be quite severe before ova are present. The double operculated eggs are distinctive. However, ova production often is sporadic and there may be few or no ova in a single fecal sample. The number of ova found on fecal examinations may not be a reliable indicator of the number of worms present.

Control

Control can depend on avoidance of exposure to contaminated pastures or lots. Tillage of pastures or lots not being used can reduce the number of eggs that survive. In outdoor operations, it is helpful to treat the pregnant sows with an appropriate anthelmintic a week or two prior to farrowing and/or before moving them to clean pasture. This reduces exposure of the piglets to eggs. Raising swine in confinement, without access to soil, usually results in good control.

Not all anthelmintics have good efficacy against *T. suis*. This necessitates a careful evaluation of a product's spectrum of activity before incorporating it into a control program. See the table, Anthelmintics and Parasiticides, on page 147.

Section IV

Nutritional Deficiencies

Nutritional Deficiencies

Iodine Deficiency (Goiter)

Hyperplastic thyroid glands (goiter) occasionally occur in swine. Goiter usually occurs as a result of one of the following: iodine deficiency in the pregnant sow; a genetic defect in the sow for the biosynthesis of thyroid hormones; ingestion by the gestating sow of goitrogenic substances (certain plants, drugs, or chemicals); or iodine toxicity from dams being fed an excess of iodine.

In swine, goiter usually occurs in iodine deficient regions where iodized salt has not been included in the dam's feed. Deficiency of iodine leads to the birth of weak or dead pigs that are largely devoid of hair. Many of the pigs have a mucinous edema, especially over enlarged foreparts of the body. The skin in these areas is thick and doughy. The tongue is often edematous and may protrude from the oral cavity. Enlarged thyroid glands (goiter) in piglets may not be visible externally but often can be palpated or observed at necropsy. In mature swine, iodine deficiency is not usually a significant disease although gestation may be prolonged by as much as seven days. Iodine deficiency is easily avoided by using iodized salt in the ration of gestating sows.

Iron Deficiency Anemia

Piglets are born with very little iron reserve. Colostrum and milk from the sow provide relatively little iron, perhaps only 15-50% of the daily requirement. Rapid growth and expansion of blood volume in suckling piglets ensures that a deficiency of iron and anemia will develop unless another source of iron is made available. This is especially the case in pigs raised in confinement without access to soil or feces containing iron. A small amount of copper is essential for utilization of iron. Copper deficiency can also lead to anemia that has many of the same clinical signs and lesions.

Signs and lesions of iron deficiency vary in piglets of different ages. Piglets not supplemented with iron will rapidly lose body condition and thrift after only about one week. At necropsy, these pigs will have pallor, a thin-walled heart, and edema of the lungs, muscles and connective tissues. In piglets that have received an insufficient supply of iron to successfully reach weaning at three to four weeks of age, rapid breathing and sudden deaths can occur. At necropsy there is marked enlargement of the heart and spleen, hydropericardium, ascites, edema in various tissues and fatty changes in the liver. Iron deficient piglets four to ten weeks of age will show similar signs and lesions. They are quite susceptible to bacterial infection and have little resistance to environmental chilling.

Diagnosis can often be made on the basis of a history that documents a lack of supplementation with iron; clinical signs and postmortem lesions will reinforce the diagnosis. Additionally, several laboratory procedures can be used to confirm the anemia. Among these is a study of stained blood smears that reveals a microcytic, hypochromic anemia. Hematology and serum chemistry will reveal reduced serum iron and transferrin saturation and a low hematocrit.

Prevention is possible by administration of supplemental iron (100-200mg). This can be done with water-soluble iron given per os or by parenteral injection of iron dextran. Parenteral administration is most commonly practiced and has the advantage of precise dosage. Iron dextran should only be injected into the neck muscles in order to prevent any possibility of staining valuable areas of the carcass. For the same reason, iron dextran should not be administered parenterally beyond seven days of age. Both forms of administration, when improperly used, can lead to iron toxicity and deaths.

Pigs deficient in vitamin E/selenium are highly susceptible to iron toxicity. Pigs raised outdoors with access to soil usually do not have an absolute requirement for iron supplementation but many producers still find it a beneficial practice even in these situations.

Parakeratosis

Parakeratosis is a zinc-responsive dermatosis usually observed in 2- to 4-month-old swine. Pigs not allowed access to soil or not supplemented with zinc are more likely to have parakeratosis. The disease is caused by a relative deficiency of zinc. The deficiency is usually caused by feeding an unbalanced diet that has one or more of the following features: excessive calcium; excessive phytic acid (sometimes present in soybean protein); or a low concentration of essential fatty acids. These features all adversely affect availability of dietary zinc. In addition, enteric pathogens or changes in intestinal flora can adversely influence zinc absorption. Parakeratosis most often is caused by consumption of excessive calcium.

Affected pigs show few signs of illness other than skin lesions and reduced growth rate. Initial lesions appear as reddened macules and papules on the ventrolateral abdomen and medial surface of the thighs; these lesions often go unobserved. The lesions are slowly covered by thick, roughened scales and crusts. More obvious lesions soon become apparent on the lower legs and on the dorsum. Lesions sometimes can be seen around the eyes, ears, snout and tail and eventually may become generalized. Affected areas of the skin are hyperkeratotic and there may be fissuring of the epidermis with secondary infection of the fissures. A unique feature occasionally seen is a focal or diffuse hyperkeratosis on the tongue. Parakeratosis is a microscopic feature of affected epidermis and gives this dermatosis its name.

Parakeratosis must be differentiated from sarcoptic mange and greasy pig disease (exudative dermatitis). Parakeratosis is nonpruritic whereas sarcoptic mange is pruritic. Greasy pig disease tends to occur in younger, smaller pigs. Pigs with parakeratosis will recover if excessive calcium is removed from the ration and it is properly supplemented with zinc. Most good commercial or carefully compounded rations now are supplemented with adequate levels of zinc salts. Although once common, parakeratosis seldom occurs today unless a feed mixing error occurs.

Rickets and Osteoporosis

Rickets is a disease of growing bones. Consequently, it usually is seen in young, weaned, growing pigs in which there is a deficiency, an imbalance, or a failure of utilization of calcium, phosphorous or vitamin D. Rickets usually is caused by a dietary deficiency of vitamin D or phosphorus. The basic abnormality is a failure of mineralization of osteoid and cartilaginous matrix, especially in growth plates. This is most obvious as a thickening and irregularity of growth plates in long bones. In confined animals not exposed to sunlight or supplemented, vitamin D may be inadequate. In pastured swine fed little or no grain or protein supplement, phosphorus may be inadequate.

Signs of rickets include poor growth, short stature, enlargement of the ends of long bones, lameness and deformation of the weight-bearing long bones. Necropsy lesions include an unusual number of recent or healing fractures, ribs that bend markedly before they fracture, and widened, thickened and irregular growth plates. Abnormal growth plates are best seen on longitudinally-sawed long bones.

Osteoporosis is a lesion of mature bones. It follows removal of much of the mineral content of the bones. It results from an imbalance between bone formation and resorption in favor of resorption. In the process there may be a softening of the bone (osteomalacia). Osteoporosis occurs often in prolific sows that mobilize minerals for high milk production. Gilts in their first lactation also are susceptible since their skeletal development may have been incomplete and there was no mineral reserve prior to pregnancy. Osteoporosis often results in fractures in the latter part of a nursing period, immediately after weaning, or during mating. Lack of exercise in confinement likely contributes to osteoporosis but inappropriate ration formulation or mixing is the most important etiological factor.

Signs of osteoporosis include lameness, recumbency, fractures and paraplegia. At necropsy, fractures often can be demonstrated in the femur, humerus or lumbar vertebrae. There may be distortions or deformities of the pelvis.

Properly balanced rations, including adequate calcium, phosphorus (in the proper ratio) and vitamin D are essential for prevention of rickets and osteoporosis. Adequate exercise also is important for normal skeletal development and maintenance. Treatment tends to be unrewarding for both rickets and osteoporosis.

Vitamin E/Selenium Deficiency

Feeds high in the concentration of polyunsaturated fatty acids, copper, vitamin A or mycotoxins can either destroy vitamin E or make it less bioavailable. Grains from soils deficient in selenium, or selenium antagonists in mixed feeds, can result in feeds low in selenium. Both vitamin E and selenium work as antioxidants.

There are three closely related, overlapping syndromes associated with vitamin E and/or selenium deficiency. The most common is mulberry heart disease (MHD). The true causal mechanism is not known but the condition can usually be prevented with additional vitamin E supplementation. MHD usually occurs when vitamin E is low but is also seen in the face of seemingly adequate levels of vitamin E in tissue or serum. MHD is manifested by sudden death in pigs a few weeks to four months of age that were believed to be in excellent health. The condition was named after the mottled appearance of the heart muscle in affected pigs. Typically, there are alternating areas of necrosis and hemorrhage throughout the myocardium. The pericardial sac is distended with fluid and fibrin strands. Straw-colored fluid is often present in the pleural cavity and lungs are edematous. Microscopically there are degenerative changes in arteriole walls at many sites. Supplementation with vitamin E, either parenterally or orally, will prevent deaths from this disease.

Hepatosis dietetica (HD) is a much more rarely encountered presentation of vitamin E and/or selenium deficiency since legal levels of selenium supplementation in livestock feed were raised to 0.3 ppm. Clinically, HD presents as sudden deaths with few or no preceding signs. This syndrome was named on the basis of hepatic lesions and the belief that they are related to the pig's diet. There are irregular focal to large areas of hepatic necrosis and hemorrhage; some lobules are distended and reddened. The gall bladder often is edematous. Myocardial necrosis and pulmonary edema may be present. Supplementation with selenium will ameliorate HD.

White muscle disease (WMD) is a presentation of vitamin E and/or selenium deficiency that is much more common in lambs, calves and chickens rather than swine. Skeletal muscle pallor or streaks of white, gritty mineralization are observed, particularly in the longissimus dorsi muscle. Microscopically, characteristic necrosis and/or mineralization of individual muscle fibers are observed.

Since these deficiencies are similar, it is not surprising that lesions of the syndromes sometimes overlap. Diagnosis can often be made on the basis of gross lesions, microscopic lesions in heart, liver, or muscles, and analysis for vitamin E/selenium levels in the liver or serum.

For prevention or treatment of a deficiency, pigs can be injected with vitamin E and/or selenium and tissue levels will be increased rapidly. Also, prevention is possible through supplementation of feed or drinking water. Sows injected in late gestation give birth to pigs with increased levels of both compounds. The syndromes described above may not always be responsive to supplemental vitamin E and selenium. MHD is more responsive to vitamin E; HD more so to selenium.

Pigs on pasture usually get enough vitamin E and selenium unless the soil is deficient in selenium. In outbreaks, feed content and quality as well as feed storage conditions should be examined carefully to determine why the feed is deficient. Improper feed storage, high copper levels, high fat levels, and poor quality feed constituents can result in destruction of vitamin E in a feed otherwise formulated adequately.

Pigs deficient in vitamin E and/or selenium may be more susceptible to other diseases. Also, deficient small piglets are quite susceptible to iron toxicity. If treated with iron dextran for anemia prevention, many deaths may occur. Myocardial lesions will closely resemble those of mulberry heart disease (MHD).

Section V

Toxicoses and Poisonings

Mycotoxicoses

Mycotoxicosis is the consequence of ingestion of grains or forage containing toxic metabolites produced by certain fungi. Fungi that produce toxins often do so only under specific conditions of warmth, moisture and humidity. Factors that adversely affect plants or their seeds (grains) often influence mycotoxin production. Mycotoxins can develop in field grains, damaged grains or improperly stored feeds.

Of the over 200 mycotoxins identified to date, at least seven have been reported to cause disease in swine. Some fungi produce more than one mycotoxin. Several different fungi can produce different mycotoxins in a single mixed feed. The toxins may be additive or may potentiate one another. When metabolized, they may be converted into other toxic substances. While toxicologic effects are numerous and often confusing, one should be careful not to implicate mycotoxins in disease processes without credible evidence.

Mycotoxins produce their toxic effects in several ways, including impairment of metabolic, nutritional or endocrine functions. Many mycotoxins damage the liver, reduce average daily feed intake, growth and feed efficiency. Some are teratogenic or carcinogenic. Some are immunosuppressive and predispose pigs to secondary diseases. Several mycotoxins decrease the reproductive performance of sows. Metabolites sometimes are passed in the milk of sows to their litters. The effect of mycotoxins may vary with the amount ingested, the time over which it is consumed, and the age of exposed swine. Young pigs usually are much more susceptible than adults. Within a herd there can be great variability in response to a mycotoxin.

Mycotoxicoses can present with either chronic or acute onsets. Most exposures are probably chronic or subacute as a result of consuming small amounts of toxin over a long period of time. In these instances, there may be few signs of toxicosis other than decreased appetite, slow growth, and increased susceptibility to secondary diseases. Acute outbreaks may have more obvious signs and will vary for each of the different mycotoxins. Diagnosis of chronic mycotoxicosis is often difficult because clinical signs are seldom overt and lesions are not specific. By the time a mycotoxicosis is considered, the suspected feed has often already been consumed with none having been collected and stored properly for analysis.

Prevention of mycotoxicosis is largely through careful selection and proper storage of high quality grains and other feed ingredients and the careful maintenance and cleanliness of feed preparation equipment. It often is worthwhile to properly dry and store samples of representative batches of grain that are used on a farm in the event they are needed for analysis later. Producers anticipating problems should locate a competent laboratory and get information on appropriate sample collection and storage techniques.

There are few, if any, highly effective treatments for most mycotoxicoses. A ration suspected of being toxic should be replaced with good quality feed. If a large quantity of the feed remains, it sometimes can be fed to less susceptible species or diluted with good quality feed so that the mycotoxin no longer is being fed at a toxic concentration. There are several mycotoxin "binders" on the market that can be used to prevent the absorption of some mycotoxin from the pig's gut.

Mycotoxins have been suggested as a cause of abortion in swine but none have shown the effect in an experimental setting. Astute practitioners should be reluctant to implicate mycotoxins as a cause of ill-defined maladies without evidence.

Aflatoxicosis

This mycotoxicosis is caused by mycotoxins produced by *Aspergillus flavus*, *Aspergillus parasiticus* or *Penicillium puberulum*. Four major toxins (B1, B2, G1, G2) are produced. B1 is of greatest significance and is a potent hepatotoxin. Fungi growing on peanuts, corn, wheat and several other cereal grains commonly produce the toxins. Maximum aflatoxin formation occurs under conditions related to the specific grain, its moisture content, storage temperature and humidity.

There is a marked age-related difference in susceptibility to aflatoxicosis. Young nursing or weaned growing pigs are much more susceptible than adults. When aflatoxin is ingested by a lactating dam, toxic metabolites are passed in her milk and serve as a source of exposure to the nursing pigs. These toxins reduce feed intake, average daily gain and feed efficiency. Since aflatoxins are immunosuppressive, signs of toxicosis often include an increase in previously controlled secondary diseases.

Acute aflatoxicosis is uncommon in swine. It is usually a subacute to chronic disease caused by daily ingestion of smaller amounts of aflatoxin over several weeks. Lesions often vary noticeably among pigs in the same affected group but are predominantly those of a hepatopathy. In the more acute cases there are sudden deaths, hemorrhages in multiple tissues, and icterus. The liver may be swollen, fatty, and have areas of necrosis. There may be a prolonged clotting time. With subacute to chronic hepatotoxicosis, the liver may be reduced in size, fibrotic, and ascites may be present.

Diagnosis is usually based on some combination of a history of slow growth (often accompanied by secondary diseases that seem unresponsive to treatment), an elevation of serum enzymes associated with hepatocellular damage, and gross lesions related to liver pathology. Microscopic hepatic lesions include bile duct hyperplasia and enlargement of hepatocytes. In swine, chronic aflatoxin toxicity can occur with at levels as low as 300 ppb in the feed; acute toxicity usually doesn't occur until concentrations beyond 1000 ppb. Aflatoxin is considered to be carcinogenic in humans.

Ergotism

Claviceps purpurea is a fungus of many grasses and several cereal grains, especially rye, oats and wheat. The sclerotium of the fungus is a dark, elongated body and often can be seen on cereal grain heads and in processed grains. The fungus produces three major alkaloids that cause ergotism. The primary lesions caused by the alkaloids include arteriolar vasoconstriction and endothelial cell injury that often leads to thrombosis. When present in low levels, the alkaloids can result in reduced growth rates. Larger amounts lead to ischemic necrosis followed by a dry, gangrenous sloughing of parts of extremities, especially tails, ears and hooves. Symptoms of ergotism are exacerbated by cold weather. In pregnant sows, ergotism can inhibit mammary development, reduce litter size, reduce birth weights, and cause a profound post-farrowing agalactia. The agalactia is believed to be related to inhibition of prolactin secretion.

Diagnosis of ergotism is based on lesions coupled with the gross or microscopic identification of significant numbers of ergot sclerotia in grains or the ground feed. Doubtful results may be verified by laboratory confirmation of significant amounts of alkaloids in the feed.

Fumonisin Toxicosis

The fumonisins include two principal toxins produced by *Fusarium moniliforme*. Signs of acute toxicity in growing and adult pigs are primarily related to the respiratory system and include dyspnea, cyanosis, weakness and death within four to ten days. Pulmonary lesions include marked pulmonary edema and hydrothorax. Pregnant sows that survive acute toxicity frequently abort in the days following their recovery. Growing pigs that survive the acute syndrome suffer from clinical signs related to a hepatotoxicosis. Their lesions may include icterus, hepatic necrosis, and megalocytosis. Differences in lesions and clinical presentation seem to be dose related.

Recent research has demonstrated that fumonisins decrease the ability of intravascular macrophages to clear blood-borne bacteria in swine, thereby potentially increasing susceptibility to respiratory disease. Fumonisin is a well known cause of leukoencephalomalacia in horses and is carcinogenic in humans at high concentrations.

Trichothecene Toxicoses

There are numerous structurally related toxic compounds produced by certain *Fusarium* species that are classified as trichothecene mycotoxins. At least three of these are of importance in pig production. Trichothecenes are cytotoxic to many cell types and are strongly immunosuppressive. Signs of trichothecene toxicity usually include feed refusal, salivation and, sometimes, vomiting. With chronic exposure there may be paresis, paralysis, or seizures. Lesions often include gastroenteritis, hemorrhagic diathesis, skin irritation, and necrosis.

Diagnosis of trichothecene-related toxicosis can be difficult. The presence of moldy or caked feed, along with a reluctance to consume it, may suggest the presence of a trichothecene toxicosis. Improvement following a change in feed suggests the original feed was contaminated.

T-2 toxin. In swine, the experimental administration of T-2 toxin, alone and with aflatoxin, has resulted in crusting and ulceration of the skin of the snout, lips, buccal commissures, and prepuce.

Deoxynivalenol (DON, vomitoxin). Deoxynivalenol is a commonly occurring mycotoxin in corn and wheat. Despite its common name of "vomitoxin," swine only rarely consume a large enough dose to produce vomiting; reduced feed intake is often the only sign present.

Zearalenone (F-2). This mycotoxin is produced by *Fusarium graminearum* and may be present in moldy corn, standing corn, other grains, and in pelleted cereal feeds. It has an estrogenic effect that results in vulvovaginitis and precocious mammary development in prepuberal gilts. Swelling and enlargement of the vulva sometimes lead to tenesmus with prolapse of the rectum. Similar estrogenic effects in gilts have occurred as a result of consuming estrogens from other sources, including alfalfa.

When consumed by nursing sows, some of the metabolites of zearalenone are passed to the offspring through her milk and can lead to estrogenic effects in the piglets, namely enlargement of the external genitalia and uterus. When the toxin is consumed by sows near the midpoint of their estrous cycles, it has a luteotropic effect and can cause persistent anestrus or pseudopregnancy. Fewer pigs per litter are born to sows given zearalenone in the preimplantation period (seven to ten days post-mating). Zearalenone, when consumed in very high doses, can cause reduced libido, decreased testicular size and preputial enlargement in young boars.

Plant and Chemical Poisonings

Cocklebur Poisoning

Cockleburs (*Xanthium spp.*) are widely distributed in the midwestern US and grow as weeds in fencerows, ditches, and low or marshy areas. The toxic principle, carboxyatractyloside, is present in the seeds and young seedlings of the plant, especially during the cotyledonary ("two-leaf") stage of growth. Seedlings may be ingested by pigs on pasture especially after spring rains when burs sprout in low-lying areas. Also, seeds may be ingested in mixed or ground feeds. Pigs may be found dead after consuming only modest number of seedlings. Because the clinical course of disease is only several hours, signs may not be observed and lesions may be absent from dead pigs. Mortality is sporadic unless plants are numerous.

In experimentally poisoned pigs, signs include depression, hypoglycemia, occasional nausea, incoordination, convulsions, and death. Lesions include serofibrinous effusions in body cavities and subcutaneous edema. There sometimes can be edema of the gall bladder wall and mild gastroenteritis. Microscopic lesions include centrilobular hepatotoxicosis with centrilobular accentuation of the liver pattern.

Diagnosis is often difficult unless cocklebur seedlings can be found in significant numbers in the pasture or seeds can be found in the feed. An "on-the-knees" search for the two-leaf stage sometimes reveals seedlings deep within lush pasture. Cocklebur poisoning must be differentiated from poisonings caused by ingestion of clay pigeons, aflatoxin, and gossypol.

In pigs showing clinical signs, mineral oil administered per os may delay absorption of the toxic principle until it can be eliminated. Injecting physostigmine has been reported to be of value in affected pigs.

Phenylarsonic (Organic Arsenical) Poisoning

Roxarsone and arsanilic acid are used to promote growth and to treat swine dysentery and eperythrozoonosis. Roxarsone is more toxic than arsanilic acid but most features of poisoning are similar in both cases. Poisoning is dose-related. Chronic poisoning may occur when low doses are given over a long period of time. Acute poisoning occurs when large amounts are consumed in a short period of time.

Signs of chronic poisoning with arsanilic acid include goose-stepping, hind limb ataxia, limb paresis, and blindness. Blindness is not typical of poisoning with other organic arsenicals. Paralyzed pigs remain alert. If provided with feed and water, they will continue to eat and drink. There are few or no associated gross lesions. Signs of acute poisoning include cutaneous erythema, ataxia, vestibular disturbances, and terminal muscular weakness. An acute gastroenteritis will often be present in these cases. Although signs and lesions of roxarsone poisoning will often be similar, an additional syndrome has been described that includes repeated convulsive seizures following exercise without the blindness produced by arsanilic acid. Microscopic lesions associated with chronic poisoning by these compounds include neuronal degeneration of optic and peripheral nerve trunks, including the sciatic nerves. Neuronal lesions may not be present in acute cases.

A tentative diagnosis can often be based on a history of misuse of the compounds and the presence of characteristic clinical signs in chronically affected swine. Diagnosis may be assisted by toxicologic assays of kidney, liver, muscle, and feed.

Prevention of organic arsenical poisoning can be achieved simply by correct management of these legal compounds during feed preparation or medication. In particular, water treated with these compounds should not be given to thirsty pigs, as they are likely to consume a toxic dose. Directions provided with the compounds should be followed carefully. The neurotoxic effect of poisoning sometimes is reversible if the compound is removed within two or three days of the appearance of signs. Blindness and long standing peripheral nerve damage may be permanent.

Pigweed Poisoning

Pigs allowed access to pastures or lots containing pigweed (*Amaranthus retroflexus*) may be poisoned.

Most poisonings occur in the late summer or fall. Signs appear within five to ten days after exposure and include trembling, weakness, incoordination, knuckling, and almost complete rear leg paralysis. Morbidity is variable; mortality can be high (75-80%) in pigs showing signs.

Lesions are those associated with acute nephrosis and heart failure. There is a marked perirenal edema. The kidneys are normal in size but may appear blanched. Other lesions include ascites, hydrothorax and edema of the ventral body wall; long-standing cases may have chronic fibrosing nephritis. Microscopic lesions in the kidneys of acutely affected pigs include necrosis of both proximal and distal convoluted tubules with numerous casts in tubules. Many glomeruli will be atrophic and have a distended Bowman's capsule containing filtrate. Diagnosis can usually be made after identification of the plants, obtaining a history of sudden access to them, and observing the clinical signs and rather unique kidney lesions. The toxic principal is not known.

There is no widely accepted treatment. Pigs should be denied access to the plants immediately, but new cases may develop for as long as ten additional days.

Salt Poisoning (Water Deprivation; Sodium Ion Toxicosis)

Salt poisoning can occur in pigs either as a consequence of water deprivation or from sudden ingestion of too much salt.

Poisoning in water-deprived pigs can occur in pigs consuming a proper level of salt but it is more likely if the salt level in the feed is excessive. Signs often are precipitated, or worsened, by allowing the pigs sudden, unlimited access to water. Water deprivation can occur for many reasons but commonly may be the result of freezing of the water source, plugged water nipples, or inadvertently leaving a water valve closed. Operators may not always be forthright in admitting human errors related to water deprivation. Poisoning has occurred following prolonged shipping without access to water, followed by unlimited access.

Following sudden heavy rains, salt poisoning can occur in swine after ingestion of salty brine from overflowing, loose-salt boxes provided for other livestock and is also reported following ingestion of whey. This type of poisoning is more likely in water-deprived pigs.

Clinical signs of sodium ion toxicosis are caused by the acute cerebral edema that occurs as a result of multiple central nervous system (CNS) lesions. Because the condition most often occurs secondary to water deprivation (rather than a primary toxic intake of salt), salt poisoning is frequently apparent at a "pen" or "herd" level. Signs include aimless wandering, blindness, deafness and head pressing. Affected pigs sometimes "dog-sit", slowly raise their nose upward and backward, and fall on their side in spasms that may be followed by paddling of the legs. They then may arise and continue their wandering.

Diagnosis associated with water deprivation may be suggested by history, signs, and elevated sodium levels in serum or cerebrospinal fluid. Gross lesions may be absent or limited to gastroenteritis. Gastroenteritis is more likely in pigs consuming salty brine and may be accompanied by diarrhea. A valuable but not infallible diagnostic aid is the microscopic observation of rather unique meningeal and cerebral perivascular cuffing by eosinophils in brain. Later and less reliably there may be laminar subcortical polioencephalomalacia or necrosis. Salt poisoning must be differentiated from all other encephalitic diseases. In an affected pen, a clue to the occurrence of water deprivation will be the absence of any urine or wet feces on the pen floor.

Water-deprived or affected pigs should be reintroduced to water slowly, given only small amounts of water at frequent intervals. This may suppress mortality. Pigs showing clinical signs usually die regardless of treatment.

Toxicities Caused by Gases

Five gases (ammonia, carbon dioxide, carbon monoxide, hydrogen sulfide, and methane) are associated with swine environments, especially confinement rearing.

Ammonia (NH_3) and hydrogen sulfide (H_2S) are normally generated from the decomposition of swine excrement. Carbon dioxide (CO_2) can cause deaths but is perhaps a lesser threat than carbon monoxide (CO) because it is heavier than air and usually only accumulates in slurry pits below pig housing and working areas. Methane (CH_4) is an explosion hazard. All five gases represent potential threats to both swine and people but ammonia, carbon monoxide and hydrogen sulfide toxicities are by far most common and are discussed below.

Ammonia Toxicity

Ammonia gas (NH_3) is formed by the decomposition of animal waste and is present at some level in most animal facilities. The odor can be detected by most people at concentrations of around 10 ppm; a level which appears to have little detrimental effect on pig health. However, when the concentration reaches 50 ppm or more, NH_3 may act as an irritant of the mucous membranes of the eyes, nasal passages, and lungs and cause ocular and nasal discharge. Concentrations of NH_3 that are high enough to be irritating to mucous membranes of pig farm workers likely have a similar effect on animals continuously exposed.

Research on swine suggests that toxic concentrations of NH_3 (over 50-100 ppm) reduce growth rate, reduce bacterial clearance from the lungs (interferes with mucociliary apparatus), exacerbate nasal turbinate lesions in pigs infected with *Bordetella bronchiseptica* and may influence the course of infectious diseases.

Carbon Monoxide Toxicity

Carbon monoxide (CO) has a much greater affinity for hemoglobin than does oxygen, effectively displacing oxygen from the blood. It combines with hemoglobin to form carboxyhemoglobin, reduces oxygen exchange, and causes mortality. Carbon monoxide is produced by incomplete combustion of any carbonaceous fuel, but most poisonings occur because of improperly functioning (yellow versus blue flame) space heaters or furnaces. Carbon monoxide is a colorless, odorless, and tasteless gas.

Recognition of malfunctioning heaters should alert one to the possibility of poisoning.

In late pregnancy sows, a high level of stillbirths and neonatal mortality is associated with CO poisoning. The sows themselves may show no other signs. Affected piglets usually show no lesions other than a pink to bright red color imparted to their blood and tissues by carboxyhemoglobin. Blood from affected piglets and fetuses with CO poisoning is usually characterized as "cherry red." The concentration of carboxyhemoglobin in fetal thoracic fluid or blood of an affected pig can be used to confirm CO poisoning.

Hydrogen Sulfide Toxicity

Hydrogen sulfide gas (H_2S) inhaled at toxic levels is dangerous and fatal to both pigs and people. The danger of high concentrations (greater than 100 ppm) of H_2S should be recognized, respected, and avoided but the usual, low level of the gas in closed confinement facilities, (less than 0.2 ppm) is not toxic and of little consequence. A "sewer gas odor/rotten egg smell" detectable by humans from 0.1 to 5 ppm, is sometimes offensive but is not toxic. Levels from 10 ppm to 100 ppm can cause eye and respiratory irritation. Humans cannot detect the odor of H2S at levels greater than 150-200 ppm because of olfactory paralysis induced by the gas. Levels greater than 200 ppm affect the nervous system; immediate collapse and respiratory paralysis occurs at levels greater than 1000 ppm.

Hydrogen sulfide is heavier than air and accumulates in liquid manure holding pits below confinement buildings. The gas usually remains dissolved in the liquid component of swine effluent and remains below the toxic level in air unless the effluent is agitated. Effluent storage pits are often agitated just prior to and during the emptying process at which time high levels of H_2S can be released. If inhaled in high concentration, H_2S can cause instant fatal systemic intoxication of exposed swine or people by directly suppressing the respiratory center in the brain. High levels of the gas paralyze a worker's sense of smell and may give a false sense of security. Workers trying to rescue affected swine or co-workers are at a very high risk of asphyxiation.

Exposure to toxic levels of H_2S can be avoided by emptying and cleaning the pit when the building is empty or when pigs and people have been moved out of the building temporarily. Adequate ventilation should be provided (fans on, curtains down) whenever pits are agitated to keep H_2S at a nontoxic level.

Section VI

Miscellaneous Lesions, Conditions, and Syndromes

Miscellaneous Lesions, Conditions, and Syndromes

Atresia Ani

The congenital absence of a patent anus at birth is rather uncommon in swine. The cause is not known but may have a genetic component or may be from an insult to the fetus in critical developmental stages in utero. The resultant megacolon may not be clinically apparent until several weeks of age.

Aural (Ear) Hematoma

These common lesions are the result of trauma to the ear followed by hemorrhage between the skin and cartilage (or within the cartilage). The subcutaneous hemorrhage resolves over several weeks to months, leaving the pinna thickened and misshapen in most cases. Trauma often is caused by bites inflicted by pen mates or by violent head shaking. Head shaking is associated with mange, infestation with lice, or feed particles in the ears. Treatment and/or drainage of the fluctuant lesion is not usually attempted or likely to be successful. Amputation of the ear is sometimes undertaken in management of severe cases.

Cystitis and Pyelonephritis

These lesions are the result of ascending bacterial infections. Various bacteria, including *Eubacterium* (*Corynebacterium*) *suis* and coliforms, have been isolated from the lesions. These lesions usually occur in older sows and are a common cause of sporadic deaths. Death often occurs during or shortly after advanced pregnancy, a time of maximum stress on kidney function. Anything that interferes with adequate water intake or urination may predispose to infection. *Eubacterium suis* is present in the preputial diverticulum of most boars. The organisms may be transmitted to the sow during copulation. Many sows with cystitis/nephritis have hematuria, the first sign of infection, within three weeks of breeding. This is followed by progressive loss of body weight. The lesions are uncommon in boars.

Dermatosis Vegetans

This hereditary defect originated in the Landrace breed. The defect can be expressed as foot deformities present at birth, or later as widely distributed expanding cutaneous lesions that involve small to large areas of skin. Skin lesions usually are apparent by the third week although some develop later. Skin lesions begin as papules and expand to form roughened plaques that soon become papillomatous. Most affected pigs die within six weeks. Many that survive have dyspnea related to interstitial pneumonia of giant cell type.

Ectopic Ossification of Mesentery

Sows and boars over three years of age occasionally are found to have ectopic ossification of the root of the intestinal mesentery. The cause of these bony spicules radiating through the mesentery is not known. Little significance is ascribed to the presence of ectopic ossification unless it is responsible for intestinal volvulus, incarceration, or accident.

Epitheliogenesis Imperfecta

This inherited condition occurs in at least four breeds and is characterized by the absence of discrete areas of skin, usually over a part of the back, loin or thigh. Lesions occasionally occur on the anterior surface of the tongue. Hydroureter and hydronephrosis commonly accompany the condition. Fetuses with extensive lesions may be aborted. Piglets born alive with extensive lesions usually die from bacterial invasion and septicemia. Minor defects may heal.

Hemorrhagic Bowel Syndrome (HBS)

This condition results in sudden death in growing and finishing pigs. Affected animals found dead are characterized by a pale, distended carcass. Necropsy reveals that the entire intestinal tract has a severely congested, thin-walled appearance. Intestinal contents are usually watery and contain unclotted brownish blood. The condition must be differentiated from gastric ulcers, gastrointestinal torsion or volvulus, and from the hemorrhagic form of proliferative enteritis. The cause is unknown. Diagnosis is made by ruling out other causes through post-mortem and histologic examination.

Hernias, Inguinal and Umbilical

Both inguinal and umbilical hernias commonly occur in swine. Inguinal hernias are believed to be inherited polygenically. The overall incidence of hernias in a normal swine population is low unless matings to a boar that transmits inguinal hernias have occurred. Inguinal hernias can be bilateral or mono-lateral with most occurring on the left side. Protrusion of intestines through the inguinal canal often follows castration of pigs that unknowingly have an inguinal hernia. If left uncastrated, strangulation of the intestine within an inguinal hernia can occur but the most significant effect of the condition is the economic discount applied to the pig at time of slaughter.

Umbilical hernias occur in both sexes and tend to develop as a result of poor umbilical cord management, navel infection, or navel sucking by penmates; the condition is not thought to be inherited.

Hydronephrosis

It is common to find large, fluid-filled cysts in kidneys of healthy swine. This incidental finding is observed during post-mortem examinations conducted for unrelated conditions or at slaughter.

Hypogalactia or Mastitis, Metritis, Agalactia (MMA)

This syndrome usually occurs within three days of farrowing and is characterized by inadequate milk production. Although hypogalactia is the most consistent sign, mastitis, fever, vaginal discharge, listlessness, weakness, anorexia, sternal recumbency and refusal by the dam to permit nursing by the piglets seem to be commonly present in affected sows. Dams usually recover within a few days to two weeks. Piglets are at high risk of dying from starvation unless cross-fostered or supplemented with other feed. Although the cause(s) is unknown, many risk factors have been associated with hypogalactia. These include lack of nursing stimulation (too few pigs or small/weak pigs), bacterial metritis, mastitis, mammary edema from errors in ration formulation, confinement with little opportunity for exercise, poor feeding management, constipation, obesity, moldy feeds, and poor sanitation in the farrowing environment.

Mastitis, often clinically undetected, is likely responsible for many cases of hypogalactia. Endotoxin from various Gram-negative bacteria, especially *Escherichia coli*, may be the basic cause of many cases of mastitis. Suppression of prolactin by endotoxin from any source results in less than normal milk production. The prevalence of MMA has decreased markedly in the last several decades with the use of modern sanitary and slatted flooring. Most problems with hypogalactia can be solved through management with careful attention to sanitation and the sow's exercise, nutrition, and body condition.

Hypoglycemia in Neonatal Piglets

Hypoglycemia is a common cause of death in neonatal piglets. Glycogen reserves are soon depleted if piglets become chilled or fail to ingest an adequate amount of milk. Chilling may occur if the effective temperature in the piglet sleeping area is less than ~95°F during the first week of life. Signs of hypoglycaemia include loss of condition, weak vocalization, faltering gait, cold skin, and recumbency. These are rapidly followed by paddling, frothing at the mouth, coma, and death if intervention does not occur. If chilling occurs, the piglets should be put in a warm environment with a supplemental heat source such as heat lamps. If the piglets are not receiving an adequate amount of milk, cross-fostering or milk supplementation can be beneficial. Porcine milk replacers, bovine colostrum, or evaporated milk diluted equally with water can be used for supplemental nutrition until piglets are able to consume nutrient-dense solid food.

Megacolon

Enlargement and dilation of the colon with feces is usually the result of rectal stricture and less frequently from colonic atony. Atresia ani leads to megacolon in pigs up to four weeks of age. Postnatal rectal strictures are a frequent sequel to rectal prolapse. Damaged rectal tissues from prolapse, whether reduced, traumatized, or chewed-off by pen mates, may heal and fibrose causing constriction of the rectum. The outcome is intermittent defecation or total obstruction of fecal flow causing the colon to dilate with accumulated feces while the pig slowly wastes away.

Colonic atony with patent rectum has been reported as a result of feeding lupine-seed meal. Neural control of tone and peristaltic movement is lost causing the colon to simply dilate with feces.

Mortality in Sows

Because of many variables affecting the quality of data collected by investigators, only generalizations can be made. Aside from infectious disease, causes of sow mortality include heart failure, cystitis, pyelonephritis, gastrointestinal problems (e.g. torsions, gastric ulcers), and complications during or shortly after parturition. Individual sow condition and housing are important risk factors as well. Currently, sow welfare issues are promoting timely individual sow assessment and intervention to decrease overall sow mortality in the swine industry.

Osteochondrosis

Osteochondrosis, also referred to as dyschondroplasia, is a generalized disease of growth cartilage. It affects most common domestic species. It often occurs in rapidly growing pigs approaching market weight or breeding age. Despite much research, the basic cause(s) is unknown but is usually related to the presence of one or more risk factors (below). The disease is characterized clinically by abnormal gait or lameness with characteristic pathologic lesions in cartilage and bone. Lesions of articular surfaces of joints include corrugations and ulcerations of cartilage, separation of cartilage from underlying bone, and development of cartilaginous cysts. Physeal cartilaginous lesions include fractures between the diaphysis and epiphysis or islands of cartilage within epiphyseal or diaphyseal bone. Lesions are often bilateral and symmetrical. Common sites of lesions in joint cartilage include the medial femoral condyle, humeral condyle, humeral head, glenoid of the scapula, distal ulna, and lumbar vertebrae. Common sites of physeal lesions include distal ulna and femur, head of the femur or humerus, and ischial tuberosity.

Dyschondroplasia has been attributed to rapid growth and early, excessive weight-bearing pressure on cartilage. Genetic background is believed to play some role. Other possible risk factors include nutritional deficiencies, flooring and housing that induce trauma, infection with *Mycoplasma hyosynoviae*, and lack of exercise. The number of pigs with lesions is often much higher than the incidence of lameness would suggest. Although some pigs recover, most affected sows are culled because of the time required for healing and the overall poor response to therapy.

Pityriasis Rosea

Pityriasis rosea is a dermatitis usually seen in four to twelve week old pigs and is characterized by 1- to 20-cm raised, reddened, ring-shaped lesions on the skin. Lesions first develop on the skin of the ventral abdomen but occasionally start in other areas. The cause is unknown. Papules first develop on the ventral abdomen and inner thighs. These early lesions expand to form circular, coalescing lesions with an expanding rim. Older lesions often have healed centers. Lesions heal in about four weeks without intervention. Pityriasis rosea is easily diagnosed by gross examination and does not require any treatment. The condition is not pruritic and seems to have no apparent effect on the health or growth rate of affected pigs. Nearly all affected pigs recover completely.

Porcine Stress Syndrome (PSS)

Porcine stress syndrome, sometimes called malignant hyperthermia or transport myopathy, is a complex, genetically transmitted myopathy usually triggered by stress or excitement. It also can be triggered by several anesthetics, including halothane, and by depolarizing muscle relaxants. Signs that appear can include tremors of the tail, back or leg muscles, muscle rigidity, inability to walk, respiratory distress, hyperthermia, blotchy dermal hyperemia, acute right heart failure, and death. Savaging of neonatal piglets by PSS-positive dams has been reported.

Postmortem lesions include early, rapid and complete rigor mortis, pulmonary edema and pale soft musculature often containing hemorrhages. Carcasses of slaughtered swine with PSS are blanched, wet and may drip excessive amounts of fluid. The meat is referred to as pale, soft, exudative (PSE) pork. Shoppers discriminate against it in the market place.

The basic abnormality is an inherited defect in the mechanism for uptake, storage and release of calcium in muscle fibers. Efforts to eliminate PSS through genetic selection have led to success in identification and elimination of a stress gene in many genetic lines but this trait is also linked to heavily muscled phenotype. A polymerase chain reaction test is widely available and used to identify hetero- and homozygous carriers of the halothane gene; both types of carrier animals should be culled.

Prolapses

Prolapse of rectal or vaginal tissues usually occur sporadically in swine but when there is a common cause, can appear as an outbreak. Although seldom seen in nursing pigs, all other age groups are susceptible.

Prolapse of the rectum is most often the result of cold stress (piling for warmth), transport stress (piling in trucks), or from severe coughing. The prolapse may also be associated with severe enteritis from any cause, especially enteritis caused by salmonellosis or ascariasis in young pigs. Other causes of the enteritis can include intestinal mycosis following prolonged use of antibiotics or chemotherapeutic agents. The feeding of whey, brewer's grains, or low fiber diets has preceded some outbreaks. Rectal prolapse can also occur as a result of severe coughing or straining caused by constipation, cystitis, vaginitis or urethral obstruction. Rectal stricture is a common sequel to prolapse of the rectum. The condition can be repaired surgically by amputation or, if the tissue is not overly traumatized, by replacement followed by use of a purse-string suture. "Rectal tubes" can also be used in repair of prolapses.

Prolapse of the vagina and/or rectum sometimes occurs as a consequence of flaccidity and relaxation of the birth canal in sows close to parturition. Prolapse of the vagina usually occurs first and is followed by prolapse of the rectum.

Zearalenone, a mycotoxin found in several feed grains, can cause vulvovaginal edema and irritation in prepuberal gilts or sows. Straining often leads to prolapse of the vagina and, perhaps, the rectum. Similar lesions can be caused by estrogenic substances in grains, certain pastures (including alfalfa) and therapeutic agents, and in products given to stimulate estrus. Genetic factors have been shown to contribute to prolapses of the vagina and uterus in some breeds.

When prolapse occurs in an outbreak situation, effort needs to be directed towards rapid identification of the triggering factor(s). Response to individual treatment of prolapse is poor with the exception of those cases identified within a few hours of their occurrence.

Pustular Dermatitis

Pustular dermatitis is usually observed only in nursing piglets. It is caused by a beta-hemolytic, Lancefield type C, streptococcal infection. Pustules appear in the inguinal area and inner surface of the rear legs but occasionally occur at other locations. The pustules soon rupture and are replaced by dark brown to black crusts. The streptococci are easily isolated from pustules. The piglets usually recover spontaneously. Recovery may be hastened by treatment with an appropriate antibiotic.

Rabies

Rabies is a highly fatal viral disease that occurs in swine bitten by an infected carrier animal. The incubation period is quite variable: nine days to four months. Clinical signs are similar to those described in other species and include sudden onset of incoordination, prostration, chewing movements, excessive salivation, inability to squeal, muscular spasms and tremors, and perhaps twitching of the nose. Death usually occurs within 72 to 96 hours of onset of clinical signs. Furious type rabies seldom occurs in swine. There are usually no gross lesions. Microscopic lesions are typical for viral encephalitis but are quite variable and inclusion bodies are often not present. Diagnosis is confirmed through fluorescent antibody staining on brain sections.

Ringworm

Ringworm (fungal infection) occurs occasionally in swine and may affect any age group. Although cases often are sporadic, occasional outbreaks affect many animals, especially sows. Most ringworm is caused by the fungi *Microsporum nanum* or *Trichophyton verrucosum*.

Lesions can occur anywhere but on older swine are usually seen on the neck or behind the ears. Ringworm lesions begin as brown expanding areas a few centimeters in diameter but eventually may enlarge to five to ten centimeters. Mature lesions have a central, brown crust; hair loss is minimal or absent and lesions are non-pruritic. In adult swine, ringworm must be differentiated from sarcoptic mange especially if lesions are behind the ears. In young growing pigs, ringworm must be differentiated from pityriasis rosea and exudative epidermitis ("greasy pig"). Diagnosis of ringworm usually can be confirmed by microscopic examination of skin scrapings or by histopathologic examination of skin lesions.

Ringworm is usually self-limiting but lesions may require months for healing to occur. Lesions are most common during the winter months. Ringworm can be treated orally with nystatin or griseofulvin but typically is left to resolve on its own. Ringworm should be considered contagious to people.

Shoulder Ulcers in Sows

Thin sows lying on hard floors in farrowing or gestation crates may develop ulcers over the spine of the scapula. Contributing factors include poor body condition, lack of adequate bedding or mats, prolonged recumbency while farrowing or nursing piglets, high humidity or wetness (often from coolers used during hot months), and reduced activity because of confinement. Lesions develop and are more severe during the three weeks after farrowing. The ulcers are the result of pressure ischemia leading to skin necrosis over the spine of the scapula. Control measures including maintaining a higher level of conditioning (fat) in sows and assuring crates are of adequate size to allow frequent repositioning.

Skin Necrosis of Piglets

Young pigs on concrete or other hard floors often develop pressure related lesions on the knees, coronets or at other sites over bony prominences. Although lesions may appear insignificant initially, they may become infected and lead to bacteremia with metastasis to joints or other sites, most frequently with *Streptococcus* spp or *Arcanobacterium pyogenes*. Losses can be substantial. Prevention is achieved through good sanitation, provision of good quality flooring materials, and use of floor mats.

Splayleg (Spraddleleg)

This abnormality of neonatal piglets is characterized by lateral extension of the hind legs with inability to adduct the legs; front legs may be variably affected. The principle lesion in affected muscles is myofibrillar hypoplasia related in part to delayed development, and in part to degenerative change.

Proposed causes or suggested risk factors include a genetic predisposition, slippery or sloped floors, porcine stress syndrome (PSS) in the parents, dietary deficiencies, and low birth weights or tremors in piglets.

If affected piglets are helped to nurse and protected from accidental injury by the sow, many will recover in one to two weeks. Tying the front legs or the back legs loosely together with sticky tape will increase the likelihood of survival. Selection of breeding stock with no tendency to produce affected litters will reduce incidence.

Sunburn and Photosensitization

Sunburn is injury to the skin caused by excessive exposure to the ultraviolet rays of sunlight. Pigs that are unaccustomed to direct sunlight may be sunburned if not exposed gradually to their outdoor environment. The white or light-colored breeds are more severely affected. Although suckling and weanling pigs are most likely to be affected, all age groups are susceptible. The ears and back get more direct exposure to sunlight and often are more severely sunburned. Sunburned skin is reddened, edematous, hot, and painful. Affected areas later appear roughened and may peel. A common clinical presentation of sunburned pigs is a brief "attack" of pain manifested as squealing or dipping the back while walking. In some cases, pigs may drop to their stomach, then get up and walk. Presumably, this is response to a feeling pain over the lumbar area. There have been reports of abortions associated with sunburn.

Photosensitization should be differentiated from sunburn. It occurs only in areas of white skin. Lesions result when pigs ingest, are injected with, or come into skin contact with a photodynamic agent and then are exposed to sunlight. Sunlight includes wavelengths that activate the photosensitization process. Photosensitizing agents are present in some pastures (alfalfa, clover, oats, rape, buckwheat, others). Also, several common pharmaceuticals (phenothiazine, tetracyclines, sulfonamides, others) may act as photosensitizing agents. The mechanism of tissue injury probably varies with the different agents.

Lesions tend to be more severe with photodynamic dermatitis than with sunburn, often resulting in exudation of serum onto the skin's surface. Exudation is followed by drying and fissuring. The lesions are pruritic. Skin necrosis with sloughing of severely affected areas often follows. Conjunctivitis, sometimes with corneal opacity and temporary blindness, may accompany photosensitization.

Pigs with sunburn or photosensitization should be kept out of sunlight. Photosensitizing agents, once identified, should be avoided.

Torsion and Volvulus

Torsions of the stomach and/or the intestines around the dorsoventral axis of the mesentery occur sporadically in pigs. Affected animals die quickly without any warning, and will appear pale and bloat very rapidly after death. There is no single, proven cause. Factors believed to contribute to torsions include: rapid ingestion of a large amount of feed or water (as with once per day feeding), overly crowded pens with associated piling and competition for feeder space, use of highly fermentable ration ingredients that produce excessive amounts of gas in the stomach or colon, and advanced pregnancy. Torsion of stomach seems more prevalent in sows that become agitated during once daily feeding. Torsion of intestine and/or colon must be differentiated from hemorrhagic bowel syndrome (HBS).

Vestibular Syndrome

A syndrome characterized by turning of the head to the affected side and a tendency to circle in that direction. The condition usually occurs in young, growing pigs. The syndrome is a consequence of either bacterial meningitis affecting the vestibular nerve or pharyngitis with extension of the infection up the Eustachian tube to the middle and internal ear. At necropsy, exudate often is demonstrable in the middle ear.

Vices (Tail Biting, Ear Biting, Flank Biting, Navel Sucking)

Tail-biting, ear-biting, flank-biting or navel sucking behavior can be serious in groups of growing pigs, particularly when confounded by secondary bacterial infections. Through careful observation, one can often identify the few individuals within an affected group that are responsible for the abnormal behavior and are inflicting trauma on numerous pen-mates. The cause of the offending behavior is too often simply ascribed to "stress." A disciplined approach is required to identify the true source(s) of the stress, which may include: facility limitations (inadequate feed or water space, overstocking), nutritional compromise (mineral or salt imbalances in rations, maladjustment immediately post weaning), environmental inadequacies (drafts, full effluent pits, temperature variation, high humidity), or management factors (co-mingling pigs, out-of-feed events, poor hygiene, concurrent infectious diseases). Control requires careful observation at two levels, first to accurately identify the offending pigs and second, to identify the risk factors that may be contributing to the aggressive behavior. It is important that the aggressive pigs be separated from the group to prevent more cases. In addition to being removed to a hospital pen environment, pigs with severe lesions will likely require systemic antibiotic therapy to prevent extension of bacterial infections locally or systemically. The administration of anti-inflammatory medication may also be warranted. Concurrently, the risk factors and potential contributors to stress should be systematically analyzed and eliminated.

West Nile Virus

This mosquito-borne *Flavivirus* can infect pigs; however, the virus does not seem to replicate in high enough numbers to permit transmission to other pigs, birds, or insect vectors. Infection is inapparent in swine and thought to occur only rarely.

Ulceration of the Pars Oesophagea (Gastric Ulcers; Ulcers)

Definition

In swine, gastric ulceration refers to the destruction of part(s) or all of the pars esophagea (non-glandular stomach) with the formation of single or multiple bleeding ulcers.

Occurrence

The lesions occur in pigs from weaning onwards; the prevalence is variable but high (5-90%) in most swine-producing areas. Clinical signs are usually only noticed in pigs eight weeks of age or older, with highest prevalence in pigs 120 pounds to market weight. Ulcers occur in all breeds, both sexes and in most major swine-raising countries.

Historical information

Ulceration of the pars esophagea (UPE) was first reported in Illinois in 1897. Subsequently, the lesion was identified in at least 30 other countries. Although the ulcers most often are subclinical, death losses have been severe enough that much research has been directed at identifying cause(s) and risk factors.

Etiology

The etiology is unknown but is likely multifactorial and represents the culmination of various permutations of any of multiple risk factors. Risk factors are largely empirical, discerned at the time animals experience higher incidence of the disease. Recently, inconsistent feed consumption associated with respiratory disease outbreaks and/or hot weather seems to be of greatest concern. Other risk factors commonly mentioned include:

- The feeding of finely ground feed (< 400 µm particle size).
- Pelleted rations, perhaps because of the finely ground feed used in making pellets.
- Concentrated, nutrient dense diets that are low in fiber.
- Stress factors (e.g. anxiety, fear, pain, fatigue, crowding, fasting, prolonged transportation, social stress from mixing with unfamiliar pigs, poor air quality, etc.) are frequently suggested.
- Greater occurrence in hot, summer months may be related to inconsistent feeding behavior or stress associated with access to water.
- Out of feed events. This may be a result of inconsistent feed availability from plugged or empty feeding systems or be the result of disease-induced anorexia.
- Greater occurrence reported in barrows (versus gilts) and in high-lean genotypes.
- Feeding rations with copper as a growth promoter, perhaps without adequate zinc.
- Ad libitum feeding of cheese whey or skimmed milk has resulted in increased prevalence.
- Diets high in wheat or cornstarch, compared to barley or milo, and/or low in protein.
- High levels of unsaturated fats in the diet, often with inadequate vitamin E.

Infectious organisms and use of non-steroidal anti-inflammatory agents and the presence of *Helicobacter pylori* are associated with human gastric ulcers that occur in glandular portions of fundus and pylorus. When pigs have been used as models for human ulcers, ulcers are induced in glandular mucosa. However, naturally occurring ulcers in pigs are in the non-glandular pars esophagea. A primary infectious etiology has not been proven nor is likely for swine. Several agents have been associated with increased prevalence and severity of UPE, including other *Helicobacter* sp. or *Gastrospirillum* sp., but a causal role has never been established. In some severe "outbreaks" of gastric ulcers in swine, porcine circovirus type 2 (PCV2) has been demonstrated within lesions. Gastric ulceration is a common sequel to outbreaks of swine influenza and porcine respiratory disease complex (PRDC), particularly during summer months.

Epidemiology

Both etiology and epidemiology are speculative. Epidemiology is difficult to assess. Risk factors that appear important in one herd or production system do not remain consistently important across others.

Pathogenesis

Irrespective of cause or risk factors, the effects are thought to be a derangement of normal gastric function. An abnormal fluid content in the stomach results in changes in the pH gradient that normally exists between the terminal esophagus and the pylorus. This results in an excessive, gastrin-stimulated acid secretion. The excessive acidity, lower than is normal at the pars esophagea, initiates changes in the stratified squamous epithelium (hyperkeratosis) that may ultimately lead to ulceration. Pre-ulcerative hyperkeratosis is extremely common in growing swine, probably because of high concentrate/low fiber diets. The pars esophagea undergoes hyperkeratosis and parakeratosis which develop fissures that expose the underlying lamina propria. If the insulting acidity persists, or animals become anorexic, part or all of the stratified squamous epithelium peels or sloughs off and leaves one or more ulcers. Blood vessels of various sizes in the lamina propria are eroded and hemorrhage begins. If blood loss is slow, melena, generalized pallor, and anemia may be observed. If a few large vessels are eroded, the animal may die from an acute massive hemorrhage. In some pigs, the ulcers may be recovered with epithelium and heal uneventfully. Occasionally, resolution of lesions results in stricture of the terminal esophagus or pars esophagea.

Clinical signs

Pre-ulcerative hyperkeratosis of the pars esophagea is common as a precursor to actual ulceration. Hyperkeratosis does not appear to influence feed consumption nor is it noticeable clinically. In fact, most swine are subclinically affected, evidenced by the high prevalence of lesions in apparently normal pigs at slaughter. Withholding feed will cause some pre-ulcerative lesions to erode in a relatively short time, as little as two to three days.

Clinical effects of ulcers are usually related to blood loss. Acutely affected pigs may be found dead with pallor. Others may have black tarry feces (melena), anemia, and generalized pallor. Other signs that sometimes can be observed include anorexia, grinding of the teeth, or unthriftiness.

Lesions

Pigs that die suddenly have pallor of the skin and internal organs and tissues. There may be large blood clots in the stomach and/or blood mixed with ingesta, throughout the intestine. The intestinal, and/or colonic contents are often very dark, black, or "tar-like." The entire pars esophagea may be eroded to muscular wall giving the false impression of intact glandular mucosa.

Ulcers typical of UPE occur only in the non-glandular region (pars esophagea) of the stomach at the junction of stomach and esophagus. Pigs that are in the early stage of developing ulcers have an altered pars esophagea which, instead of being snowy white, is raised, roughened, somewhat nodular, usually bile stained, and sometimes fissured with hyperkeratosis. Ulcers vary greatly in size, shape, number and depth. Large ulcers often are deep and have smooth, rolled and raised borders. Sometimes the ulcerated area involves the entire pars esophagea and may partially obstruct the esophagus. The terminal part of the esophagus may also be hypertrophied. In animals that have recovered from deep ulcers, a puckered or stellate scar often remains. Complete destruction of the pars esophagea is easy to miss at necropsy; the color of that area may be a uniform gray and without hemorrhage. The absence of clotted blood in the stomach does not rule out UPE; careful examination of the pars esophagea is warranted since hemorrhage may be intermittent. Death caused by UPE does require a large amount of clotted blood to be found in the stomach at the time of death.

Differential diagnoses include other causes of hemorrhagic diarrhea such as porcine proliferative enteritis, swine dysentery, salmonellosis, or whipworms.

Control

Pigs suspected of having ulcers should be separated from the herd. If pale or anemic, treatment may include Vitamin K and hematinics, although treatment is of questionable efficacy. Access to fiber (hay, pasture) will sometimes aid in recovery.

Prevention is based on correcting those risk factors suspected of contributing to ulcer formation (see under Etiology). Minimizing stress and preventing out of feed events via consistent feed availability/delivery is always warranted. Altering the ration to minimize the effects of some of the possible risk factors is helpful. Changing to a more coarsely ground feed (>700 microns), including changing from a pelleted diet to a meal diet, is often recommended. The quality of the feed ingredients should be improved if some of the feedstuffs were stored for long periods or of poor quality. Successful control of swine respiratory diseases, especially swine influenza, has decreased the losses attributable to UPE on some swine farms.

Section VII

Exotic Viral Diseases

African Swine Fever

Definition

A highly contagious, viral disease with signs, lesions and other features that closely resemble classical swine fever (CSF). The disease is exotic to the US.

Occurrence

African swine fever (ASF) occurs naturally in wild, feral and domestic swine (*Suidae*). At present, ASF does not occur in the western hemisphere. It is endemic in several African countries and an outbreak of the disease has been occurring across several countries in Central Asia since 2007. Distribution among countries changes, depending on new infections, re-infections and the success of eradication programs.

Historical information

African swine fever first was described in Africa in 1921. It soon was endemic in eight African countries. In 1957, the disease occurred in Portugal, the first non-African country to be infected. Over a 28-year period, ASF spread to eight European countries, Brazil, Cuba, Haiti and the Dominican Republic.

In some countries, repeated outbreaks have discouraged eradication efforts. In many other countries, eradication efforts have been successful. Prohibiting importation of swine and pork from infected countries, and eliminating or regulating the practice of waste-food feeding to pigs are fundamental to most successful eradication programs. Several features of ASF, plus the high cost of eradication, make worldwide eradication unlikely. The United States has never experienced an outbreak although ASF has occurred several times in nearby Caribbean islands.

Etiology

Formerly classified as a member of the Iridoviridae, this DNA virus is currently the only member of a family called Asfarviridae. Strains vary markedly in virulence and no effective vaccines currently exist. It grows readily in several cell culture systems. ASF virus is exceptionally hardy in the environment but can be inactivated by many disinfectants.

Epidemiology

The virus often is introduced by feeding uncooked garbage containing scraps of infectious pork. ASF virus persists in pork for long periods of time. Once the virus is introduced, direct or indirect contact of healthy swine with it leads to outbreaks. Most outbreaks can be traced to contact with infected swine. African swine fever can be transmitted by direct contact with infected animals, indirect contact on fomites, and by tick vectors. Direct transmission usually is through oronasal secretions.

In many endemically infected countries, several species of soft ticks (predominantly genus *Ornithodorus*) act as reservoirs and vectors. In Africa, a cycle of inapparent infection is established between ticks and wild boars, warthogs and bush pigs. ASF virus is passed transovarially in some ticks and persists in successive generations of ticks. Difficulty in eradication of ticks interferes with eradication of ASF. The United States has ticks with a similar potential.

Pathogenesis

The primary infection usually starts in the tonsils and mandibular lymph nodes. Virus then spreads in lymph and blood to secondary replication sites (bone marrow, lung, spleen and kidney). A persistent viremia begins about one week after infection. The main target cells of the virus include monocytes, macrophages, cells of the reticuloendothelial (RE) system, endothelial cells, and platelets. Destruction of antigen processing cells in lymph nodes, spleen and bone marrow apparently interferes with formation of protective antibodies. Destruction of endothelial cells and vascular damage is responsible for hemorrhages, edema and transudate formation. The virus also causes a meningoencephalitis responsible for ataxia. The virus affects multiple organs of fetuses and causes fetal deaths.

Clinical signs

Clinical signs appear five to fifteen days after infection. Signs vary greatly, depending on the virulence of the virus, and can range from inapparent or subclinical to hyperacute with sudden death. Many initial outbreaks are acute and closely resemble outbreaks of acute CSF.

In acute outbreaks, signs include anorexia, high temperatures, listlessness, incoordination, leukopenia, cutaneous hyperemia, hemorrhages on the skin (especially on ears and flanks), and hyperpnea. Vomiting, diarrhea, dehydration and ocular discharge may occur. Morbidity and mortality are high and can approach 100%. Death usually occurs in four to seven days. In subacute or chronic cases, signs include abnormal respiration, abortion and low mortality.

Lesions

The lesions are similar to those of CSF. There are petechial and ecchymotic hemorrhages at many sites (skin, kidneys, lymph nodes, serosal and mucosal surfaces, epicardium, endocardium, larynx, bladder, gall bladder, lung), edema, hydrothorax, hydropericardium and ascites. The liver and spleen are congested. The spleen often is enlarged, friable, and may have infarcts. There often is congestion of meninges and brain. Lesions that are often present with ASF, but seldom with CSF, include hydrothorax, hydropericardium, ascites and pulmonary edema. Hemorrhages and edema usually are more severe than with CSF.

Gross lesions in chronic cases of ASF include fibrinous pericarditis and pleuritis, spleen and lymph node enlargement, caseous lobular consolidation of areas in the lungs, possibly with mineralization.

Histologic lesions of ASF include meningoencephalitis, periportal hepatitis, extensive necrosis with karyorrhexis (cell nucleus rupture) in lymphoid tissues, and degeneration and necrosis of endothelial cells and cells of the mononuclear-phagocytic system.

Diagnosis

Diagnosis can be made by detecting ASF virus, viral antigen, or antibodies to ASF. A hemadsorption test is widely used to identify the virus. Viral antigen can be identified in tissue by direct immunofluorescence on frozen sections and is widely used. Also, several techniques have been developed to identify ASF virus in paraffin-embedded tissue sections. Several tests are used to identify ASF antibody. These include indirect immunofluorescence, enzyme-linked immunosorbent assay (ELISA), complement fixation (CF), immunoblotting and radioimmunoassay. There is a sensitive dot immunobinding assay for field diagnosis.

Control

Control in most countries is limited to preventing entry of the ASF virus. Early diagnosis of suspected cases is important. State and federal disease control authorities should be informed immediately if an ASF or CSF outbreak is suspected. If ASF should gain entrance, early quarantine and restriction of movement of animals in the area are important. Vaccines are unsatisfactory both for control of clinical signs and preventing infection.

Massive amounts of virus are found in many tissues especially blood. Care must be taken when performing necropsies to prevent substantial environmental contamination.

Cooperative international laws prohibit the importation of swine and pertinent food products from countries where ASF is endemic. Most countries prohibit the dumping of food wastes from planes and ships.

Should outbreaks occur in the US, they probably will be handled by slaughter, followed by cremation or burial of infected pigs and pigs that had direct or indirect contact. Strict restriction of animal movement in the area, cleaning and disinfection of premises and the use of sentinel pigs prior to repopulation will also be necessary.

Blue Eye Disease (Paramyxovirus)

Definition

Blue eye disease (BED) is the common name for a disease caused by a porcine rubulavirus (Paramyxoviridae; La Piedad Michoacan virus) that is characterized in nursing or growing pigs by central nervous system (CNS) signs and, frequently, by corneal opacities. Signs in sows and boars include various forms of reproductive failure and corneal opacity.

Occurrence

Blue eye disease is only known to occur in swine. In Mexico, the only country that has reported cases, BED occurs throughout the year but is more common in the hotter, drier months (March to July). Swine diseases caused by other paramyxoviruses have occurred in several countries (Japan, Israel, Canada, United States, and Australia) but the diseases they cause are sporadic, rare, and are distinctly different from BED manifesting as transient outbreaks of pneumonia, encephalitis, or reproductive disease.

Historical information

Blue eye disease first occurred in 1980 in a large swine raising operation in central Mexico. Within a short time it had spread to eleven other states or districts and had become economically important. The first outbreaks occurred mainly in unweaned piglets less than 30 days old, frequently in piglets less than two weeks old. After 1983, severe outbreaks occurred in larger pigs (33-99 lb). Signs of reproductive failure were also observed in mature sows and boars. The scarcity of reports since 1990 suggest BED is less common now.

Etiology

The agent that causes BED is a paramyxovirus. It grows in chick embryos and hemagglutinates erythrocytes of mammalian and avian origin. It grows and causes cytopathic effect in PK-15 and several other cell culture systems. It stimulates formation of inclusion bodies in PK-15 cells. Formalin destroys infectivity of the virus.

Antisera against seven paramyxoviruses and six parainfluenza viruses do not affect infectivity of the BED virus. This suggests BED virus differs from other paramyxoviruses and causes a unique disease in swine. Other paramyxoviruses are infrequent causes of swine pneumonia and encephalitis.

Epidemiology

Subclinically infected pigs are the main reservoir of virus. Virus can also be disseminated by people and vehicles. On farms with a continuous production system, virus persists and is maintained in new groups of susceptible young pigs while adult stock remains well. The disease is largely self-limiting in closed herds. Infected animals develop protective antibodies that usually persist throughout their lifetime.

Pathogenesis

Natural infection is thought to occur by inhalation based on experimental exposures where intratracheal and intranasal exposure reproduced the disease. The initial site of viral replication is unknown but may be in the nasal mucosa or tonsils. Virus soon spreads to the brain, lung and many other organs, suggesting that viremia occurs. Reproductive problems in dams suggest that the virus crosses the placenta and infects the fetuses.

Corneal opacities (blue eye) sometimes occur late in the course of the disease. The opacities disappear spontaneously, presumably as inflammatory edema resolves. The opacities are, perhaps, the result of an immunologic reaction accompanied by inflammation. Virus may replicate in the eyes since inclusion bodies have been demonstrated there.

Clinical signs

Signs vary somewhat with the age groups affected but are mainly those of encephalomyelitis in both young and growing pigs. In young piglets, onset is sudden with prostration and fever. Other signs include ataxia, weakness, muscle tremors, rigidity, nystagmus, abnormal postures, hyperexcitability, squealing, and paddling movements; occasionally there is blindness. Often there is conjunctivitis with adherence of the eyelids. Corneal opacity (blue eye) may occur in 1-10% of young piglets and may be seen in the absence of other signs. Twenty to 65% of litters can be affected. Morbidity within litters is between 20-50%; mortality in affected pigs can reach 90%. Piglets affected early in an outbreak often die within 48 hours; those affected later usually die after a course of four to six days. Mortality occurs over a two to nine week period.

In pigs greater than 30 days old, signs are more moderate and transient. They include fever, sneezing, coughing and anorexia. CNS signs include listlessness, ataxia and circling. Less than 5% of the pigs are affected and mortality usually is low. However, in pigs weighing 35 to 45 lb, outbreaks with 20% mortality and up to 30% corneal opacity have occurred. Adult animals occasionally develop corneal opacities.

In pregnant swine, returns to estrus may occur and persist in the herd for six to eight months. There also is an increase in stillbirths and mummified fetuses, and occasional abortions. In affected boars, there is a reduction in fertility and an increase in testicular size, usually unilateral, followed by atrophy.

Lesions

Gross lesions are limited and largely nonspecific. They may include mild anteroventral pneumonia, tonsillitis and mild ascites with some fibrin. Brain congestion and an increase in cerebrospinal fluid may be present. There is conjunctivitis and, perhaps, corneal opacity in one or both eyes. Pericardial and renal hemorrhages also have been reported. In affected boars there is orchitis, epididymitis and testicular atrophy.

Microscopic lesions include a nonsuppurative encephalomyelitis affecting mainly the gray matter of the midbrain, thalamus and cerebral cortex. Intracytoplasmic inclusions in neurons have been reported. Affected eyes have corneal edema and anterior uveitis, perhaps with exudate in the anterior chamber. Intracytoplasmic inclusions may be present in epithelial cells near the drainage angle of the corneoscleral junction.

Diagnosis

Clinical signs of encephalomyelitis, along with corneal opacity, suggest a diagnosis of BED. Reproductive problems in either or both sexes, along with numerous corneal opacities, are also suggestive. Microscopic lesions of encephalomyelitis and the presence of intracytoplasmic inclusion bodies in neurons or eyes strongly suggest BED.

The hemagglutinating virus usually can be isolated from the brain or tonsil in PK-15 cells and can be identified by hemagglutination inhibition (HI), virus neutralization (VN) or enzyme-linked immunosorbent assay (ELISA). The HI test is widely used. Direct immunofluorescence has been used to identify the virus in cell culture. BED must be differentiated from other causes of CNS disease, especially pseudorabies.

Control

A rigorous health control program to prevent introduction of virus is the best preventive measure. Maintaining a closed herd and use of the all in/all out system of production may be helpful. Essential replacement stock should be added only after negative serologic tests and a period of quarantine. Commercial vaccines have been produced but there is no report on their efficacy.

BED has been eliminated from infected sites by disposing of infected animals, cleaning and disinfecting the site and using sentinel pigs to confirm elimination of infection. There is no satisfactory treatment of BED and pigs with CNS signs usually die. Pigs having only corneal opacities frequently recover without treatment.

Classical Swine Fever (Hog Cholera)

Definition

Classical swine fever is a highly contagious, viral disease of swine that in its most virulent form causes morbidity and mortality approaching 100%. Viral strains of low to moderate virulence cause infections with a gradient of severity, some clinically inapparent.

Occurrence

Classical swine fever (CSF) occurs only in swine, and all age groups are susceptible. The disease occurs in most major swine-raising countries where eradication programs have not been successfully implemented. In the United States, CSF was once a frequent occurrence but was eradicated in 1976. Classical swine fever currently exists in many countries, including areas of Central and South America and the Caribbean, which present nearby threats to the US. Since 1997, epidemics of CSF have been reported in many European countries, including The Netherlands, Spain, Germany and Italy. Sporadic outbreaks continue to occur, particularly in Eastern Europe. The disease is endemic in much of Asia.

Historical information

The historical record does not clearly indicate where CSF originated. A disease now believed to have been CSF occurred in Tennessee in 1810 and in Ohio in the early 1830s. Subsequently, CSF was reported from many other countries throughout the world. Classical swine fever has been eradicated from at least ten countries, but remains persistent in much of the world.

In the United States, there were many years when CSF was epidemic and caused huge losses. Losses were first reduced through vaccination with CSF antiserum/virus (serum/virus). When properly done on healthy swine, it resulted in strong immunity but was accompanied by several disadvantages. As examples, vaccination sometimes triggered outbreaks of other diseases and vaccinated swine commonly shed virus that could serve as a source of infection for other herds. Some of the later, attenuated vaccines had similar disadvantages. Vaccination with serum/virus or attenuated vaccines was prohibited as part of a national eradication program begun in 1962. This, along with other measures, resulted in eradication of CSF by 1976. Eradication was a remarkable achievement, considering the highly infectious nature of virus and extensive commerce in pigs and pork products.

Etiology

Classical swine fever is a *Pestivirus* (family Togaviridae), related to the virus of bovine virus diarrhea (BVD) and sheep's border disease (BD). Strains of CSF vary greatly in antigenicity and virulence. Virulence can increase in a single passage through pigs. Strains of high virulence cause classic outbreaks with high morbidity and mortality. Strains of moderate virulence cause subacute or chronic infections. Strains of low virulence can cause mild or inapparent infection, reproductive failure or neonatal losses.

CSF virus is moderately resistant to environmental influences. In pig houses, excreta and bedding, virus can persist for days to weeks, depending upon temperatures. The virus survives some curing processes as well as in frozen pork for months to years, and in chilled meats for months. The virus is inactivated by 2% sodium hydroxide or by lipid solvents.

Epidemiology

Classical swine fever is highly contagious and infection spreads rapidly by direct or indirect contact between infected and susceptible pigs. Pigs with acute infection shed large amounts of virus before they are visibly ill, during illness, and after recovery. Live pigs infected as fetuses spread virus in their secretions and excretions. Uncooked waste food containing infectious pork scraps and subsequently fed to pigs has been well documented as initiating many outbreaks. Other methods of viral spread include farm equipment (contaminated wagons, trucks, tractors, machinery), personnel (careless farmers, salesmen, veterinarians), fomites, pets, birds and arthropods. Airborne transmission probably is of little significance.

Pathogenesis

After ingestion, the virus infects epithelial cells in the crypts of tonsils, spreads to adjacent lymph nodes and produces viremia within 24 hrs. Tonsils are the initial site of viral replication. Replication also occurs at other sites, especially in lymphoid tissues (spleen, Peyer's patches, lymph nodes, thymus), in endothelial cells, bone marrow and circulating leukocytes. Within three to four days, virus spreads to many epithelial-type cells and is present in excretions and secretions.

The virus causes lymphoid depletion which makes the swine more susceptible to other infections. Bone marrow damage leads to leukopenia and thrombocytopenia. Thrombocytopenia, along with endothelial cell damage, results in petechial and ecchymotic hemorrhages at many sites. Swine with chronic CSF infection may develop glomerulonephritis from antigen-antibody complexes that damage glomeruli.

In pregnant sows and gilts, the virus may cross the placenta and infect some or all of the fetuses. The effect depends on the stage of pregnancy and can include abortion or production of mummified fetuses, stillborn piglets, or persistently infected live piglets. Fetal anomalies may result from in utero infection; a remarkable one is hypomyelinogenesis, a syndrome that results in shaking piglets (myoclonia congenita).

Clinical signs

In typical acute outbreaks, clinical signs are nonspecific. These include: depression (a hunched posture with drooping head and a straight-hanging tail), anorexia, high fevers (106° F), conjunctivitis, and a strong desire to lie down and huddle or pile with other affected pigs. There may be diarrhea or constipation, and perhaps vomiting. Signs caused by central nervous system (CNS) lesions often are apparent and include reeling when forced to walk, eventual hindquarter paresis or paralysis and occasional tonic/clonic convulsions in young growing pigs. Most affected pigs die within three weeks of onset.

Outbreaks with less virulent virus or chronic cases seldom present with typical signs but often have conjunctivitis, diarrhea or constipation, and some degree of emaciation. Mildly virulent strains of the virus seem to be becoming more prevalent worldwide and present a significant opportunity for misdiagnosis by those veterinarians and producers unfamiliar with the disease. Pigs infected as fetuses or neonates may present no signs.

Lesions

In typical acute CSF, lesions include petechial and ecchymotic hemorrhages at several common sites including the epiglottis, bladder mucosa, cortex and pelvis of the kidneys, gall bladder mucosa, on the lungs and heart, at the ileocecal junction and in the skin. Lesions sometimes considered of special value in diagnosis include single or multiple infarcts along the border of a spleen of normal size, subcapsular hemorrhage in many lymph nodes, and hemorrhages on the cortices of the kidneys and on the lungs. There usually is some degree of congestion in the fundus of the stomach and small intestine. Small foci of necrosis may be present in the tonsils.

Peracute cases may have no lesions. In chronic cases, ulcers with raised edges ('button ulcers") are often present in the cecum and/or colon. Grossly visible fetal lesions include ascites, hepatic nodularity, pulmonary hypoplasia, petechiation of the skin, microencephaly, hydrocephalus and cerebellar hypoplasia.

Microscopically, there is a panencephalitis more apparent in the medulla, pons, midbrain or thalamus. Glial cell nodules often cluster around destroyed capillaries. Vascular lesions are present at many sites, perhaps more pronounced in splenic follicular arteries.

Diagnosis

Typical acute CSF should be suspected on the basis of history, clinical signs, temperatures and gross lesions. Numerous postmortem examinations will increase the accuracy of diagnosis. Leucopenia in several suspected cases is suggestive of CSF. The lesions of typical, acute cholera closely resemble and must be carefully differentiated from those of African swine fever, acute salmonellosis and acute swine erysipelas. Lesions sometimes resemble those of other septicemic diseases, including streptococcosis and Glasser's disease. Infection with mildly virulent strains may be indistinguishable from many endemic systemic or respiratory pathogens. Diagnostic testing is imperative whenever the combination of gross pathology, clinical signs, and response to therapy suggest that CSF is on the list of possible etiologies.

Suspected outbreaks should be immediately reported to authorities to confirm diagnosis. Three laboratory procedures commonly used are: demonstration of CSF viral antigen in frozen tissue sections by immunofluorescence with preferred tissues being tonsil, pharyngeal lymph nodes, spleen, kidney and distal ileum; isolation of virus in cell culture and identification of viral antigen in the culture by the fluorescent antibody (FA) test; and identification of antibodies to CSF by virus neutralization tests. Regardless of the procedure used, it may still be necessary to differentiate CSF from BVD. A monoclonal antibody technique is available.

Control

Control is possible through prevention of exposure, vaccination, or eradication. In most countries, prevention of exposure is attempted through banning/controlling importation of live pigs, fresh pork, insufficiently heated pork products, and other possible sources of virus (imported swine semen and embryos, biologics); and prohibiting the feeding of uncooked waste food and the dumping of garbage from ships in port.

In countries where the virus is endemic, attenuated vaccines often are used for preventing or reducing the prevalence of infection. A strain of virus attenuated by passage in rabbits (C strain) is widely used. Vaccination may be prohibited when eradication by slaughter is introduced. In the final stages of eradication, infected and exposed swine are slaughtered and buried or incinerated. Movement of swine in the area is controlled. Contaminated facilities are disinfected and not repopulated for a period of time.

Bovine viral diarrhea virus (BVDV) and border disease virus (BDV) of sheep

These two diseases and classical swine fever (CSF) are closely related members of the family Togaviridae. Naturally occurring infections with BVDV and BDV have occurred in swine. Their major importance in swine is that they both induce antibodies that can lead to serologic misdiagnosis of CSF. This can cause confusion in countries trying to eradicate CSF or maintain a CSF-free status. This confusion can be avoided if specific laboratory methods of CSF diagnosis are used.

Clinically apparent outbreaks of BVDV and BDV in swine are uncommon. Outbreaks that have been suspected are manifested in breeding herds as reproductive problems, such as poor conception rates, small litters, abortions, and an excessive number of dead and mummified fetuses. In infected, live piglets, the signs are expected to be similar to those of congenital CSF including deaths in piglets less than five weeks old, anemia, unthriftiness, congenital tremors and convulsions.

Foot-and-Mouth Disease (FMD)

Definition
Foot-and-mouth disease (FMD) is a highly contagious viral disease of many wild and domestic cloven-footed mammals and many other animals. In swine, the disease is characterized by vesicles on the feet, snout and in the mouth.

Occurrence
A wide range of wild and domestic animals, especially cloven-footed mammals, are susceptible to FMD. Horses are resistant, a fact useful in differential diagnosis. The disease occurs in most countries with a large livestock population unless those countries have eradicated it and maintained their disease-free status. In countries where FMD occurs endemically and pigs are present in large numbers, swine frequently are infected. All age groups are susceptible.

Historical information
Foot-and-mouth disease is an ancient disease. A description of a disease observed in 1546 probably is a description of FMD. Since FMD was first clearly delineated from other diseases, it has continued to cause major losses in livestock throughout the world. Losses have been greater from loss of productivity than mortality.

Nine outbreaks of FMD have occurred in the United States. All outbreaks were followed by eradication, often at great expense. Much of the livestock population now in the United States is highly susceptible. An outbreak of FMD could cause great loss, especially if the outbreak became widespread before it was recognized. The United States has remained free of FMD since the last outbreak in 1929.

Recent outbreaks in Asia and the UK have demonstrated the devastation and frustration wrought by FMD. Exports were embargoed and entire regional herds slaughtered, effectively destroying the swine industry in these countries.

Outbreaks of all vesicular diseases of swine are of concern because the lesions cannot be distinguished from those of FMD, except by laboratory means. Swine are of special concern because they are susceptible to more vesicular diseases than other species of livestock, and they often play a major role in the spread of FMD by producing large, infectious aerosols of virus.

Etiology
An *Aphthovirus* of the family Picornaviridae causes FMD. There are at least seven immunologically distinct types of virus: A, O, C, South African Territory (SAT) 1, 2, 3 and Asian 1. Among the seven types, one particular antigen (virus infection-associated antigen [VIA]) is group reactive and useful in serologic diagnosis of FMD infection.

Over 60 subtypes of virus have been identified and new subtypes continue to develop. Many differ enough antigenically to require preparation of subtype vaccines for their control. The antigenic variation of the virus and the limited cross protection among strains has made it impossible to prepare a single vaccine that protects satisfactorily against all strains. Effective disinfectants of FMD virus include sodium hydroxide, acetic acid, sodium carbonate and Virkon® (Durvet).

Epidemiology
Virus transmission occurs through respiratory aerosols and direct or indirect contact with infected animals. Aerosol transmission of FMD virus over distances as great as 30 miles is believed to occur under certain weather conditions. Infected swine are exceptional disseminators of virus. For some virus subtypes, they are able to produce aerosols many times greater in virus concentration than those produced by cattle or sheep. They are sometimes referred to as "amplifier hosts" for FMD virus.

Infected swine disseminate virus in their excretions and secretions. Food products containing infectious pork can also spread FMD virus. Virus persists for long periods of time in frozen meat products. In several notable FMD outbreaks, the index case has been associated with the consumption by pigs of uncooked waste food containing infectious meat scraps. Contaminated biologics, including vaccines, have been responsible for outbreaks. People with residual FMD virus in their respiratory tract can transmit the virus to livestock for a short time.

Some species of animals recover from FMD and remain carriers for weeks, months and possibly, years. Occasionally they disseminate virus that initiates new outbreaks. Swine are not believed to be long-term carriers of FMD virus.

Pathogenesis
Foot and mouth disease virus adheres to the mucosa of the respiratory tract, the usual site of virus entry. Macrophages are believed to transport virus to secondary sites that include epithelium, mucosa and myocardium. In secondary sites, the virus replicates, then a marked viremia develops and the virus infects epithelium at many other sites. Within a few days vesicles develop, usually at sites of mechanical stress. In swine, common vesicle sites include the snout, mouth, tongue, and especially the feet. In cattle, the FMD virus affects the mammary gland epithelium and virus is shed in milk for a prolonged period. Although unproven, similar shedding may occur in swine.

The lesions of the major vesiculating viral diseases are similar. Vesicles develop in the epidermis, and the epithelium over the vesicle soon sloughs. Enough of the stratum basale is preserved to regenerate the epidermis unless there is secondary infection of the lesions. Secondary infection occurs on the feet of some swine and leads to chronic lameness.

The FMD virus often causes severe myocardial necrosis in neonatal and young pigs. This often leads to sudden deaths from myocardial failure. The mottled myocardial lesions sometimes are referred to as "tiger-heart" lesions and are useful in diagnosis.

Clinical signs

An incubation period of one to five days precedes clinical signs. Lameness is often the first sign noticed. There is an initial acute rise in temperature; slobbering and chomping are common signs. Pregnant sows may abort or deliver stillborn, infected pigs. Sudden deaths may occur in neonatal pigs, sometimes before signs or lesions are apparent in the sow. The early stages of lesions appear as blanched, small foci in the skin on the snout, soft tissues of the feet, and perhaps the teats of lactating sows. By the time signs are readily apparent, there are usually cutaneous vesicles or bullae. Signs develop rapidly and morbidity rapidly increases. Mortality usually is less than 5% but there can be higher mortality in young pigs.

Lesions

Well-developed vesicles and bullae are soon apparent. They are frequently present on the snout, behind the rim of the snout, in the nares, on the tongue and lips, and on the soft tissues of the feet, including the coronary band, the bulbs of the toes and interdigital clefts. Lesions probably are more common on the feet than in the mouth. Less often the lesions are on the vulva, the teats of lactating sows, or the scrotum of boars. Extensive lesions on the coronary band may lead to sloughing of the hoof and lameness. Foot lesions may involve one or more of the feet. Vesicles usually rupture within 24 hours and the superficial epidermis sloughs to reveal hyperemia and hemorrhage on underlying tissue. Uncomplicated lesions usually heal within two weeks. In a virulent form of FMD, young pigs, and sometimes older animals, may have extensive mottled areas of myocardial necrosis on ventricles and in papillary muscles.

Diagnosis

Diagnosis cannot be made reliably on the basis of clinical signs and lesions since they are similar in all the vesicular viral diseases of swine. The state veterinary office should be contacted immediately if an outbreak is suspected. Differential diagnosis of vesicular viral diseases should only be completed in specifically-designated laboratories having specific arrangement to safely handle exotic disease organisms. Plans must be made for collecting and mailing specimens. The Foreign Animal Disease Diagnostic Laboratory (FADDL), Plum Island, NY, often does the diagnostic work.

Diagnostic techniques used include serologic tests to identify FMD virus infection-associated antigen (VIA), complement fixation (CF) and enzyme-linked immunosorbent assay (ELISA) tests to detect FMD viral antigen, virus isolation (VI) and neutralization (VN), electron microscope (EM), and animal inoculation studies. Polymerase chain reaction (PCR) tests have been developed and are frequently utilized. FMD must be differentiated from all other vesicular viral diseases and from other diseases that cause erosive/ulcerative lesions in the oral cavity. Positive diagnoses usually require less time than negative diagnoses. An ELISA is available that can differentiate antibody titers from infected versus vaccinated animals but is not yet officially recognized by many countries.

Control

In the United States, prevention of FMD depends on regulations that govern the importation of animals, animal products, semen, embryos, and on regulations related to the safety of vaccines and other biologic products. There are special regulations on both cooking and dumping of waste food to prevent spread of the virus. Reliance on the vigilance of veterinary practitioners and diagnostic laboratory personnel is important in early detection of outbreaks.

In countries where FMD has not been eradicated, vaccines are used for prevention. The recently developed subunit vaccines have been of value in preventing some types and subtypes of FMD infection but have not provided consistent protection for type O infection, the most prevalent form of FMD. In the event of an outbreak in the United States, vaccine use will be considered but control is anticipated to occur primarily through slaughter of infected animals. The disease will be managed through quarantine, restriction of movement of animals in quarantined areas, slaughter followed by burial or incineration of infected and exposed animals and disinfection of production sites. Eradication is considered to be less costly than living with FMD.

Japanese B Encephalitis

Definition

Japanese B encephalitis is an exotic, mosquito-borne disease affecting many animals, including wild birds, horses, swine and people. In swine, the only evidence of disease may be reproductive failure.

Occurrence

Japanese B encephalitis (JE) occurs in most domestic animals; also in wild birds, reptiles, perhaps chickens, and people. Swine can be infected and all ages are susceptible. Major epidemics have occurred in horses, donkeys and people.

Japanese encephalitis is confined largely to southeastern Asia, Indonesia, and major Pacific islands. At least 20 countries have reported occurrence of the disease. In many locales, epidemics correlate with the mosquito season.

Historical information

Japanese encephalitis was first described in 1933. Major epidemics in people have been reported from Japan, Korea, India and Nepal. The disease has not been reported in the western hemisphere. Abortion in women, and encephalitis in children, have been caused by JE so the virus is recognized as an important zoonosis.

Etiology

The etiologic agent is a single-stranded RNA *Flavivirus* and is related to West Nile virus. It is unstable in the environment and easily inactivated by many disinfectants. The virus can be grown in many cell culture systems, including cells derived from embryonic or larval mosquito tissues.

Epidemiology

Mosquitoes become infected by feeding on viremic hosts. The virus is then transmitted through the mosquitoes' saliva when they subsequently feed on uninfected people or animals. The virus is transmitted mainly by mosquitoes of three genera (*Aedes*, *Culex*, and *Anopheles*) and can be transmitted vertically in some species of mosquitoes. Infected mosquitoes feed on a wide range of mammals, birds and reptiles. Infected pigs become viremic and are a major source of virus for mosquitoes. Often there is a correlation between outbreaks in people and the concurrent presence of infected mosquitoes and swine in the region. Other known or suspected reservoirs include snakes, lizards, many wild birds and chickens.

Pathogenesis

Infected pigs remain viremic for several days. On the basis of research largely in other animals, the virus is believed to induce suppressor T-cells to produce a factor that suppresses humoral and cell mediated responses. This makes animals less resistant to infection. In porcine fetuses, the virus often causes the development of anomalies in the brain as well as encephalitis and degenerative neuronal changes.

Transplacental infection in swine sometimes occurs. The effect of the virus depends on whether the fetuses are immunologically competent. When dams are infected between 40-60 days in gestation, fetuses often are killed and some are mummified. There may be no effect on fetuses if they are 85 or more days in gestation. Fetal deaths are believed to be caused by destruction of vital stem cells.

Clinical signs

Mature swine seldom show signs of infection other than those of reproductive failure. Signs may occur in fetuses or piglets if their dam was infected during pregnancy. Signs include stillborn and mummified fetuses or weak pigs that may have signs of central nervous system (CNS) disease. Subcutaneous edema and hydrocephalus may be present in stillborn pigs. Abortions seldom occur. Infected boars may have orchitis, reduced libido and disturbance of spermatogenesis. Young, susceptible pigs occasionally contract JE and show signs of CNS lesions.

Lesions

Gross lesions in stillborn or weak, infected piglets include hydrocephalus, subcutaneous edema, ascites, hydrothorax, hemorrhages on serous membranes, congestion of lymph nodes and necrotic foci in the liver and spleen. Other lesions may include congested meninges, hypoplastic areas in the cerebral cortex, hypoplasia of the cerebellum or spinal hypomyelinogenesis.

Histologically, in infected fetuses or piglets there is diffuse nonsuppurative encephalitis, neuronal degeneration and necrosis in the cerebrum and cerebellum. In mature boars there is excessive fluid in the tunica vaginalis, orchitis, epididymitis, and degenerative changes in seminiferous epithelium.

Diagnosis

A definitive diagnosis is often based on isolation and identification of the virus from fetuses or infected piglets. Virus usually is isolated from brain extracts inoculated into suckling mice or cell cultures. Virus can be identified by neutralization tests in suckling mice or cell culture. Alternatively, viral antigen in tissues from infected fetuses or stillborn pigs can be identified by fluorescent antibody (FA) or avidin-biotin staining using formalin-fixed tissues treated with trypsin. In suspected outbreaks, serial serum samples from pigs sometimes are used to show a rising titer against JE. Serologic tests that reveal antibody in fetuses also are useful in diagnosis.

Control

It may be possible to break the cycle of infection by controlling mosquito populations, but this often is impractical. The disease can be controlled by vaccinating the breeding stock; vaccines are common in parts of Asia. Young gilts and boars are vaccinated twice at two to three week intervals prior to the mosquito season. Growing pigs are also vaccinated in endemic areas.

Porcine Epidemic Diarrhea

Definition
A coronavirus causes this exotic viral diarrhea of swine that closely resembles transmissible gastroenteritis (TGE).

Occurrence
Porcine epidemic diarrhea (PED) occurs only in swine. In previously unexposed herds, all age groups are susceptible. The disease occurs in England, many European countries, China, Taiwan and Korea. Thus far the disease has not occurred in the western hemisphere.

Historical information
In 1971, outbreaks of watery diarrhea in feeder and fattening swine were observed in England. Suckling pigs did not sicken; otherwise, outbreaks closely resembled TGE. In 1976, a similar disease, but also affecting suckling pigs, was observed. Eventually the two diseases were referred to as PED type 1 and PED type 2.

During the 1980s a similar disease with two virulence types was prevalent in many European countries. Also, PED spread to China, Taiwan and Japan. In Europe, outbreaks now are rare, usually affect feeder and fattening pigs, and are not economically important. The disease in Asian countries, however, is highly virulent. Efforts there are under way to develop an oral vaccine for immunization of sows.

Etiology
A coronavirus causes porcine epidemic diarrhea. The virus is unrelated to porcine coronaviruses that cause TGE, porcine respiratory coronavirus (PRCV) and hemagglutinating encephalomyelitis virus (HEV). It does have some antigenic determinants in common with feline infectious peritonitis virus. The virus can be grown in epithelial cells from the mucosa of the small intestine of hysterectomy-derived piglets and in Vero cells. Porcine epidemic diarrhea virus induces antibodies in swine that can be identified by various laboratory techniques.

Epidemiology
Coronavirus is disseminated in the feces of infected pigs for at least seven days post-inoculation. Fomites and vehicles can also spread virus indirectly. There is little information on the possible existence of carrier swine that could spread virus. On sites where PED is endemic and there is frequent or continuous farrowing, virus is maintained in successive generations of susceptible piglets.

Pathogenesis
The coronavirus of PED, like that of TGE, is in feces and usually is transmitted orally. It replicates primarily in enterocytes on villi of the small intestine, and to a lesser degree in cryptal cells of both small intestine and colon. In the small intestine, it causes degeneration and necrosis of enterocytes. Many enterocytes are destroyed and replaced by cuboidal or flat epithelial cells. Intestinal lesions of PED are similar to those of TGE but develop less rapidly and are less severe. Erosion and ulceration of enterocytes leads to loss of tissue fluid into the lumen and failure of the intestine to absorb adequate fluids. Diarrhea follows and leads to dehydration and depletion of electrolytes.

Clinical signs
The main sign in all age groups is watery diarrhea. The disease closely resembles TGE but spreads more slowly than TGE on a site and among adjacent farms. Infected piglets up to one week old die from dehydration after three to four days. Mortality averages about 50% but usually is lower than that of TGE. Older piglets recover in about one week. In other outbreaks, weaned pigs and older animals are severely affected but younger animals may not sicken and have little or no diarrhea. The severity of disease is quite variable.

Feeders, finishers and adult swine have diarrhea, depression, anorexia, and signs of abdominal pain. Outbreaks often start in these age groups. Morbidity may be high and affected animals are quite sick. Although recovery usually follows, there may be some mortality and occasional sudden deaths.

Lesions
In piglets with PED, there usually are few gross lesions other than dehydration and a distended intestine filled with yellow fluid. In fattening hogs that die suddenly, there may be extensive necrosis of back muscles, a unique lesion. Microscopically, villi in the small intestine of piglets are atrophic. Some villi are fused with adjacent villi or poorly covered with cuboidal to flattened epithelium.

Diagnosis
When all age groups are affected, a firm diagnosis cannot be made on the basis of clinical signs. Signs closely resemble those of TGE although PED spreads more slowly. A diagnosis of PED may be suggested by failure of baby pigs to become ill when adult animals are sick. Necrosis of back muscles in older swine is suggestive.

Diagnosis sometimes can be made after direct immunofluorescence tests on cryostat sections of the small intestine of acutely infected young pigs. The test is both rapid and reliable. It identifies virus or viral antigen in affected epithelial cells. In older, acutely infected animals, an enzyme-linked immunosorbent assay (ELISA) test on feces or intestinal content may be used to detect viral antigen. Direct electron microscope (EM) examination of feces may be helpful in identifying a coronavirus but does not differentiate PED from TGE because the viruses have similar morphology.

Several serologic tests can be used to demonstrate rising antibody titer to PED. Paired serum samples should be taken, the first at the onset of diarrhea and the second no sooner than four weeks later. Antibodies persist for at least one year.

Control

There are no vaccines available. Pregnant sows more than two weeks away from parturition can be intentionally exposed in the face of an outbreak. This can be done by feedback of watery feces or intestinal content from acutely affected pigs. This procedure has the obvious risk of spreading other diseases.

Sanitary and quarantine measures may slow the spread of PED. There is no effective treatment other than good care and the provision of adequate water to combat dehydration.

Vesicular Exanthema of Swine
(San Miguel Sea Lion Viral Disease)

Definition
In swine, an acute, contagious disease caused by a *Calicivirus* and characterized by vesicles on the feet, snout, mucous membranes of the mouth and tongue, and non-haired skin. The disease in sea lions causes vesicles on the flippers.

Occurrence
Of the domestic animals, vesicular exanthema (VE) occurs only in swine. The disease has only occurred in the US; in swine shipped from the United States to Hawaii, and in swine fed raw garbage from a US military post in Iceland. The disease has never been reported from any other country. Vesicular exanthema has not recurred in domestic swine since it was eradicated in 1956.

San Miguel sea lion viral disease (SMSL) occurs in sea lions, fur seals, elephant seals, opal-eye fish and several other marine animals of the western coast of the United States.

Historical information
Beginning in 1932, a vesicular disease, now believed to have been VE, occurred repeatedly in California. The lesions closely resembled those of foot-and-mouth disease (FMD). Outbreaks were contained by slaughtering the infected herds. In 1951, uncooked garbage from a train originating in California was fed to swine in Wyoming. Those swine developed vesicular exanthema. The disease spread throughout many states. Eradication required five years. In 1959, VE was declared to be an exotic disease.

Beginning in 1973, caliciviruses indistinguishable from the virus that causes vesicular exanthema were isolated from sea lions, northern elephant seals, fur seals and certain kinds of fish. Each of the viruses can produce lesions in swine and certain sea mammals.

Etiology
The calicivirus that causes VE and SMSL is believed to be the same. However, spontaneous outbreaks of VE in swine caused by SMSL virus have not been substantiated. Caliciviruses have a cup-shaped morphology from which they are named. The calicivirus that causes VE is sensitive to many common disinfectants including 2% sodium hydroxide.

Antibodies to several other closely related caliciviruses have been detected in both marine and terrestrial animals. The latter include swine, cattle, donkeys, foxes and buffalo. The taxonomy and exact relationship between these various caliciviruses have yet to be agreed upon.

Epidemiology
The opal-eye fish (*Girella nigricans*) now is believed to be the primary host of the calicivirus that may be passed to pinnipeds and swine. The method of spread of the virus among sea lions and other sea mammals is speculative. It could be through ingestion of infected fish or small marine life, by coastal contamination, or direct contact.

Swine usually are exposed to the VE calicivirus by eating uncooked garbage containing infectious meat scraps from swine or certain fish. Although unproven, some marine origin feed supplements for swine may contain calicivirus. Vesicular exanthema is quite contagious among swine and spreads by direct contact and fomites. Neither long-term carriers nor aerosol spread have been demonstrated.

Pathogenesis
In swine, the VE calicivirus is ingested in uncooked garbage. Virus enters the epithelium through abrasions and multiplies in the basal layer of the epidermis. Intracellular and intercellular edema and coalescence of disintegrating cells leads to vesicle formation. Virus spreads cell to cell as lesions develop. A low-grade viremia occurs and leads to secondary lesions at other sites. Extensive lymphocyte destruction occurs in regional lymph nodes. Since much of the basal layer of epidermis survives, regeneration of epithelium in swine usually occurs within one to two weeks. Lesions in sea lions closely resemble those seen in swine.

Experimentally, it requires much more virus by oral exposure to produce VE than is required by intradermal injection. This suggests that the virus can be spread more readily through abrasions on the skin.

Most swine with VE probably would recover if allowed to do so. However, it is required that they be destroyed as a precaution to prevent the surreptitious entry of foot-and-mouth disease.

Clinical signs, lesions, diagnosis and control
See Foot-and-Mouth Disease and Vesicular Stomatitis on pages 137 and 77. These aspects of the various vesicular viral diseases of swine are similar. See the table, Vesiculating Viral Diseases, on page 163.

Section VIII

Tables

Anthelmintics and Parasiticides for Swine

Agent	Common name	Products					
		Piperazine	Pyrantel	Avermectins	Levamisole	Dichlorvos	Fenbendazole
Stephanurus dentatus	Kidneyworm	–	–	+	+	–	+
Haematopinus suis	Lice	–	–	+	–	–	
Metastrongylus spp.	Lungworm	–	–	+	+	–	+
Sarcoptes scabiei	Mange mite	–	–	+	–	–	–
Oesophagostomum spp.	Nodularworm	+	+	+	+	+	+
Ascaris suum	Roundworm	+	+	+	+	+	+
Macracanthorhynchus hirudinaceus	Thorny-headed worm	–	–	–	–	–	–
Stonglyloides ransomi	Threadworm	–	–	+	+	–	–
Trichuris suis	Whipworm	–	–	–	+	+	+

Arthritis in Young Pigs and Associated Etiologic Agents*

Diseases and agent	Age group affected	Nature of lesions	Signs, other lesions, comments
Mycoplasmal polyserositis/ arthritis *Mycoplasma hyorhinis*	3-10 weeks. Occasionally in young adults.	Swollen joints, serosanguinous or serofibrinous synovial fluid. Later, perhaps pannus and joint erosion.	Acute onset and lameness, fibrinous pericarditis, pleuritis, peritonitis singly or in combinations. Abdominal tenderness with sternal recumbency. Morbidity <25%, mortality usually low.
Mycoplasmal arthritis *Mycoplasma hyosynoviae*	8-24 weeks.	Excessive serosanguinous joint fluid. Later, yellow membranes, perhaps pannus.	Stiffness, shifting lameness. Hind leg lameness common. Many slowly recover. Morbidity 1-50%, mortality low.
Glasser's disease *Haemophilus parasuis*	Pigs from 2 weeks to 4 months old. Occasionally in young adults.	Swollen, painful, fluctuating joints with turbid fluid or green fibrin. Periarticular inflammation.	Classic lesions: serofibrinous or fibrinopurulent pleuritis, pericarditis and peritonitis or combination. Frequently meningitis and convulsions. Often affects best pigs.
Streptococcal arthritis *Streptococcus suis* Type 2	In weaners and growers up to market weight.	Acute suppurative polyarthritis. Meningitis common.	If meningitis, then CNS signs. Often fatal in weaners and growers. Can be epidemic with incidence up to 15%. Occasionally, valvular endocarditis.
Streptococcal arthritis *Streptococcus equisimilis*	Suckling and postweaning pigs.	Hot swollen joints. Increased turbid synovia. Perhaps periarticular fibrosis, abscesses.	Accompanied by fever, depression and other evidence of septicemia. Endocarditis occasionally in older pigs.
Erysipelas *Erysipelothrix rhusiopathiae*	Young growing, weaned pigs. Also in finishers with acute erysipelas.	**Growers:** joint(s), especially hocks, knees, toes are swollen, painful; joint(s) decrease in size but remain enlarged. **Finishers:** limited swelling, severe pain.	**Grower:** Number of swollen points in herd increases, often without an acute outbreak or much mortality. **Finishers:** Acute arthritis often a part of acute erysipelas. Identify erysipelas by culture of parenchymatous organs and acutely inflamed joints.
Septic arthritis Other bacteria	Neonates to piglets a few weeks old.	One or several painful, swollen joints.	Commonly caused by metastatic bacteria from infected navel, skin erosions/ulcerations at other sites.

* Joints of knees, hocks, toes more visibly affected. Also examine shoulder, stifle, atlanto-occipital joints. Culture joints, parenchymatous organs.

Key: CNS-central nervous system

Clostridial Diseases

	Species Affected*						Major Toxins				
TYPE**	**Sw**	**Sh**	**Go**	**Po**	**Ca**	**Ho**	**ALPHA**	**BETA**	**BETA-2**	**EPSILON**	**IOTA**
CptA	X	X		X	X		X		X		
CptB		X			X	X	X	X		X	
CptC	X	X	X	X	X	X	X	X			
CptD		X	X		X		X			X	
CptE		?			X		X				X

* Sw=swine Sh=sheep Go=goats Po=poultry Ca=cattle Ho=horses

** CptA= *Clostridium perfringens* type A; CptB = *Clostridium perfringens* type B, etc.

Diarrheal Diseases

Disease and agent	Groups affected	Diagnostic features and methods
Enteric colibacillosis *Escherichia coli*	Neonates one day old to pigs up to 2-4 weeks postweaning.	Watery diarrhea, possibly vomiting. Minimal lesions; jejunum and ileum may have mild villous atrophy. Many Gram-negative rods on mucosa. Culture uniform population of *E. coli* from small intestine. Identify enterotoxigenic *E. coli* enterotoxins(s) and/or pili, usually by PCR. *E. coli* may also cause fibrinous polyserositis.
Rotaviral enteritis (Rotavirus, usually group A)	Usually 1-6 week old piglets. Also common about one week after weaning.	Diarrhea, occasional vomiting. Usually nonfatal. Variable enteritis with moderate villous atrophy. Identify rotavirus in feces of early cases by EM or ELISA or in small intestinal epithelium by FAT or IHC.
Transmissible gastroenteritis (TGE) Coronavirus	All age groups susceptible if previously unexposed. Most severe in piglets <4 weeks old.	**Acute form:** vomiting and very high mortality in piglets <3 weeks old. Bright yellow feces often seen in older piglets. Marked diarrhea in feeder age pigs. Acutely infected sows may vomit, are depressed and refuse to nurse piglets. **Endemic form:** similar signs but much less severe and with reduced mortality. FAT or IHC on intestine of acutely affected pigs or PCR on feces from acutely affected pigs.
Clostridium difficile-associated enterotoxemia	Piglets 2-10 days of age with diarrhea, variable morbidity and low mortality	Mesocolonic edema and colon filled with creamy diarrhea. Microscopically, there is multifocal suppurative and erosive colitis. The presence of *C. difficile* enterotoxin is confirmed by ELISA test on fresh feces.
Clostridium perfringens type A-associated enterotoxemia	Piglets 2-10 days of age with diarrhea, variable morbidity and low mortality	Minimal gross lesions, similar to colibacillosis. Microscopically there is mild multifocal suppurative enteritis with large Gram-positive rods. Isolation and genotyping of an enterotoxigenic (beta 2 toxin) *C. perfringens* type A is warranted.
Salmonellosis Usually *Salmonella* serotypes Choleraesuis, Typhimurium, or Heidelberg Other salmonellae are commonly isolated but primary role in disease is often unclear.	More common in weaned and growing pigs. All ages susceptible if previously unexposed.	**Intestinal form:** Necrotizing enteritis of large and small intestine. Enlarged mesenteric lymph nodes. Congested lungs. Chronic cases may have rectal strictures or "button ulcers" in large intestine. **Septicemic form:** Red/purple skin lesions on ears, tail, snout, feet, abdomen. Congested lungs, splenomegaly and hepatomegaly. Perhaps gray foci in liver. **Diagnosis:** Severe septicemia or necrotizing enterocolitis. Culture Salmonella from lymph nodes, liver, lungs, spleen, kidneys, perhaps brain if CNS signs. **Histology:** Paratyphoid nodules in liver.

Diarrheal Diseases (continued)

Disease and agent	Groups affected	Diagnostic features and methods
Swine dysentery *Brachyspira hyodysenteriae* Previously *Serpulina* or *Treponema*	From 3 weeks to adults if previously unexposed.	Mucohemorrhagic diarrhea (fresh mucus and fresh blood) is very suggestive. Mucohemorrhagic to fibrinonecrotic typhlitis and colitis but no lesions in small intestine. **Histology:** Lesions largely restricted to mucosa with organisms in epithelium and crypts. Culture *B. hyodysenteriae* from mucosa or feces. **Note:** *Brachyspira pilosicoli* is a sporadic cause of colitis.
Proliferative enteritis *Lawsonia intracellularis*	Weaned pigs and all older swine.	**Signs:** Subclinical disease with weight loss most consistent sign. Clinically affected have either an acute form with hemorrhagic diarrhea or chronic form with diarrhea and wasting. **Lesions:** Thickening of mucosa of jejunum and/or ileum and/or colon. Curved bacilli in affected enterocytes. PCR (feces) and IHC (lesions) confirm organism and disease.
Whipworm infection *Trichuris suis*	Feeder/finishers and mature swine	Mucoid or mucohemorrhagic diarrhea with loss of condition is suggestive. Inflammatory nodules, often with protruding parasites, in mucosa of large intestine. Signs similar to those of swine dysentery and they can occur together. No eggs apparent until 8 weeks post-infection. Early cases diagnosed by histopathology or mucosal scrapings.

Key: CNS-central nervous system; ELISA enzyme-linked immunosorbent assay; EM-electron microscopy; FAT-fluorescent antibody; IHC-immunohistochemistry; PCR-polymerase chain reaction

Diarrheal Diseases at Various Ages

Infection with and/or agent	Unweaned piglets	Nursery pigs	Grow/finish pigs	Adults
Enterotoxigenic *E. coli*	++++	+++	+ (early grower)	
Rotaviral infection	++++	+++	+ (early grower)	
Transmissible gastro-enteritis virus (TGE)	++++	+++	+++	+++
Clostridium difficile	++++			
Clostridium perfringens Type A	++++			
Clostridium perfringens Type C	++++	+ (rare)		
Coccidiosis *Isospora suis*	++++	++	+	
Salmonellosis	+	++	++++	+
Swine dysentery *Brachyspira hyodysenteriae*	+	++	++++	++
Proliferative enteropathies *Lawsonia intracellularis*		++	++++	++
Porcine epidemic diarrhea virus (exotic)	+++	+++	++++	++++
Whipworm infection *Trichuris suis*		++	++++	+++

Key: Clear cells indicate groups that seldom, if ever, are infected; 1+, 2+, and 3+ indicate increasing frequencies of infection, with 4+ indicating the age groups that most often are infected.

Diseases Associated with Central Nervous System (CNS) Signs*

Disease	Agent	Clinical signs	Diagnostic aids and comments
Edema disease	Certain serogroups (genotypes) of (usually hemolytic) *E. coli*	Onset often within 2 weeks of weaning. Ataxia, incoordination, mental confusion, recumbency, perhaps edema of eyelids, face, nose or lips. Most die within two days. **Chronic:** Head tilt, incoordination, unthriftiness.	Edema, if present, a useful lesion. At necropsy, edema in stomach wall and spiral colon in some. Culture gut for hemolytic *E. coli* and genotype isolate for shiga-like toxigenicity. Chronics may have encephalomalacia in brain stem.
Teschovirus infections	Teschovirus	Most outbreaks in Europe; **Teschen Disease:** High morbidity and mortality in all age groups. Ataxia leading to paralysis. Opisthotonus, convulsions, nystagmus, coma, death. **Talfan Disease:** Similar but less severe and only in young pigs. In US, posterior paralysis occasionally seen.	Isolate and identify serotype. Histopath lesions and their distribution are suggestive of diagnosis. In the US, few highly pathogenic strains but most herds have endemic infections of low virulence.
Hemagglutinating encephalomyelitis	Coronavirus	**Piglets < 4 weeks:** Vomiting, retching, dehydration, wasting, coma, death. **Encephalitic form:** Same, followed by tremors, hyperesthesia, dog-sitting, walking backwards, nystagmus, convulsions, recumbency, paddling with legs, bloating, coma, death. Mortality can approach 100%.	Isolate and identify virus from brain of early, acute case. Histopath of value. Serial blood samples may show rising titers to virus. Many herds in the US endemically affected but outbreaks are uncommon.
Phenylarsonic compound (organic arsenic) poisonings	Arsanilic acid and roxarsone	**Acute:** Convulsions following exercise; incoordination progressing to paraplegia. No blindness. **Chronic:** Ataxia and incoordination leading to paralysis. Blindness if from arsanilic acid.	Signs and history of overmedication or misuse often adequate for diagnosis. **Histology:** Demyelinating lesions of cord and peripheral nerves are suggestive. Prompt analysis of kidney, liver, urine and ration may identify excessive levels.
Pseudorabies (PRV) Aujeszky's disease	Herpesvirus	**Neonates < 3 weeks:** Incoordination, ataxia, salivation, opisthotonus, seizures, recumbency with paddling. Sudden death common. **Older pigs:** Similar but less severe signs. Naïve growers/finishers/adults: respiratory signs or abortions. CNS signs may occur sporadically and vary in severity.	Consider signs in all age groups and area history of disease. Virus isolation and identification from tonsil, brain, spleen, liver, lung, cervical nodes. A reportable disease with national/state/industry eradication program.
Streptococcal meningitis	*Streptococcus suis*	**Weaners/growers:** Incoordination, tremors, opisthotonus, convulsions, blindness, deafness.	Culture brain and cerebrospinal fluid. Identify the organism. Histopath of brain is helpful. Polyarthritis, myocarditis and pneumonia often present. May be endemic in herd.
Water deprivation (Salt poisoning)	Sodium toxicity (Too much salt; or water deprivation)	Acute onset, many affected. Aimless wandering, blindness, deafness, dog-sitting, convulsions, prostration with paddling, coma, death.	History of water restriction or deprivation followed by unrestricted access. Ration can have normal levels of salt. **Diagnosis:** Histopathology and chemistry of the brain.

* Other less frequent association of CNS signs include acute classical swine fever in young growing pigs, CNS metastases of pasteurellae, *E. coli, Haemophilus parasuis, Salmonella* serotypes, also viral infection including rabies, and toxicities (organophosphate, carbamate, chlorinated hydrocarbons). Male Landrace and Landrace-cross piglets and British Saddlebacks of either sex sometimes have a genetic defect that may result in CNS signs.

Diseases Associated with Hemorrhage in Intestine*

Disease	Ileal lesions	Severity of lesions in cecum/colon	Enlargement of ileocecal nodes	Other features that may occur and comments
Salmonellosis	Mild	+++	+++	Pneumonia, hepatic foci, rectal stricture.
Swine dysentery	Usually absent	++	++	Mucohemorrhagic feces common.
Ileitis	Proliferative, hemorrhagic or necrotic	++ Lesions can be restricted to proximal cecum/colon	+++	Ileum often rigid and hose-like. Cases often sporadic in herd.
Hemorrhagic bowel syndrome (HBS)	Transmural congestion of intestine with unclotted blood in lumen	Colon may have blood contents	Sometimes edema in lymph nodes	Cause unknown; must be differentiated from intestinal volvulus.
Gastric ulcers	Dark, tarry blood in intestine or colon	No mucosal lesions in intestine or colon	Lymph nodes normal	Hemorrhage may be intermittent, therefore blood may not be present in stomach. One must examine the pars oesophagea for ulceration.

* These diseases usually are seen in grower pigs. Other enteric diseases occur but usually are in younger, smaller pigs.
Key: ++ = Mild, +++ = Marked.

Internal Parasites

Common and/or scientific names of parasitism and parasite	Usual location and gross length	Intermediate hosts or direct cycle	Mode of infection	Treatment*
Ascariasis *Ascaris suum*	Small intestine, bile ducts, stomach 15-30 cm	Direct	Orally from contaminated environment	All
Coccidiosis *Isospora suis*	Small intestine	Direct	Orally from contaminated environment	None
Eperythrozoonosis *Mycoplasma suis*	On erythrocytes 0.8-1.0 μm	Intermediate hosts. Possible direct	Arthropod bites? Contaminated instruments?	Tetracyclines Arsenicals
Kidney worm infection *Stephanurus dentatus*	Adults in perirenal fat, kidneys, ureters walls. Juveniles in ectopic sites. 20-45mm	Earthworms. Also direct	Larvae in earthworms. Prenatally, orally; skin penetration by juveniles	FBZ, AVE, LVM
Lungworm infection *Metastrongylus* spp.	Posterior border of diaphragmatic lobes of lungs. 20-50 mm	Earthworms. Also direct	Ingest larvae or earthworms with encysted larvae.	DCV, FBZ, AVE
Thorny-headed worm infection *Macracanthorhynchus hirudinaceus*	Small intestine, usually ileum Up to 30 cm	Direct	Prenatally, transcolostrally, orally, cutaneously	None
Threadworm infection *Strongyloides ransomi*	Small intestine of suckling pigs 3.3 -4.5 mm	Direct	Prenatally, transcolostrally, orally, cutaneously	DCV, FBZ, AVE, LVM, TBZ
Whipworm infection *Trichuris suis*	Cecum and large intestine 5-8 cm	Direct	Ingestion of embryonated ova	DCV, FBZ
Gullet worm *Gongylonema pulchrum*	Subepithelium of esophagus, tongue	Dung beetles	Ingestion of beetle with encysted larvae	FBZ, AVE, LVM
Red stomach worm *Hyostrongylus rubidus*	Stomach < 10 mm	Direct	Ingestion of larvae	DCV, FBZ, AVE, TBZ
Thick stomach worms *Ascarops strongylina* and *Physocephalus sexalatus*	Stomach	Dung beetles	Ingestion of beetles with encysted larvae	FBZ, DCV
Hookworm *Globocephalus urosubulatus*	Small intestine of feral and pastured swine in southern US	Direct	Larvae bore into skin	DCV, FBZ, AVE, LVM
Liver flukes *Fasciola hepatica*	Liver of pigs on pastures used by sheep. 30 mm	Snails	Ingestion of encysted metacercariae on grass	None
Trichinosis *Trichinella spiralis*	Muscle of many mammals, especially swine and bears	Many mammals	Ingestion of muscle with encysted larvae (raw garbage, wild animal carcasses, rats, mice, cats) or cannibalism	Not practical
Pork measles *Taenia solium* (a tapeworm of man)	*Cysticercus cellulosae* in skeletal and cardiac muscles of swine. < 18 mm	Swine	Ingestion of human feces containing gravid proglottids	None

Key: DCV=dichlorvos, FBZ=fenbendazole, AVE=avermectin, LVM=levamisole, PIP=piperazine, PRT=pyrantel tartrate, TBZ=thiabendazole.

Mycoplasma-Related Diseases

Name of the mycoplasma	Name of disease	Signs and lesions	Diagnosis and comments
Mycoplasma hyopneumoniae	Mycoplasmal (Enzootic) Pneumonia	**Age:** 6 weeks to market age (especially 2-4 month old pigs) **Clinical:** persistent, dry cough and dyspnea with flare-ups of pneumonia. Good appetites but unthrifty. **Lesions:** Cranioventral lobules of clearly demarcated gray consolidation, mucopurulent exudate in airways. Morbidity variable/mortality low. Histologically there is marked lymphoid hyperplasia around airways.	Often diagnosed on the basis of signs, lung lesions at necropsy and slaughter. IFAT of lung lesions may reveal mycoplasmas. Difficult to culture. Serology (CF, ELISA, and IHA) is sometimes used for herd diagnosis. Improved housing and ventilation with reduced stocking density help in control.
Mycoplasma hyorhinis This organism can be found in association with various lesions in swine but a primary role in disease is unclear.	Mycoplasmal Polyserositis and Arthritis	**Age:** Usually in 3-10 week old pigs but sometimes in young adults. **Clinical:** Acutely affected pigs visibly ill and with fever. Abdominal tenderness with preference for sternal recumbency. **Lesions:** Serofibrinous pericarditis, pleuritis and peritonitis. Later there may be fibrous adhesions. Arthritis often severe in one or more joints; later, villous hyperplasia, possibly pannus.	Isolation of the organism from acute cases. Morbidity 20 to 35% but mortality low. Infection may persist in joints but many lame pigs slowly recover with internal adhesion and poor gains. Differentiate from *Haemophilus parasuis* and *Streptococcus suis*.**
Mycoplasma hyosynoviae	Mycoplasmal Arthritis	**Age:** In pigs 12-24 weeks old. **Clinical:** Lameness, difficulty in arising, kneeling in some. Often in straight legged, muscular pigs with hidden joint swellings. Serofibrinous exudate with synovial membranes swollen.	History, signs and lesions are suggestive. May respond well to lincomycin, tylosin, or tetracycline injection. Isolate organism from acutely infected joints. Differentiate from *Haemophilus parasuis* and *Strep. suis*, erysipelas.**

Key: IHA-indirect hemagglutination; FA-fluorescent antibody; ELISA-enzyme-linked immunosorbent assay; CF-complement fixation; IFAT-immunofluorescent antibody test

* Many other mycoplasmas have been isolated from swine but these three are the only ones clearly identified with disease.

** *Haemophilus parasuis* and *Streptococcus suis* cases often have arthritis and/or synovitis and a fibrinous meningitis. Meningitis usually is absent in the mycoplasmoses

Reproductive Failure - Considerations when Farrowing Rate is Low

Conception failure (Regular returns to estrus)

- Accumulation of repeat breeders

Primary failure

- Management
  - Number of matings/services
  - Mating quality
  - Timing of mating
  - Type of service
    - Natural vs AI
    - Homospermic vs Heterospermic
- Gilt/sow factors
  - Farrow interval
    - Lactation length
    - Weaning to service interval
  - Mycotoxins
  - Parity
  - Reproductive disease
    - Systemic
    - Urogenital
  - Temperature
- Boar factors
  - Age
  - Disease
  - Genetics
  - Individual differences
  - Season
  - Temperature
  - Number of matings

Pregnancy failure (Irregular returns to estrus)

Gilt/sow factors

- Diseases
  - Reproductive
  - Non-reproductive
- Endocrine dysfunction
  - Primary
  - Zearalenone
- Parity

Feed

- Mycotoxins
- Feed additives
- Micronutrients
- Energy intake

Environment

- Temperature
- Season
- Housing
- Movement and commingling

Reproductive Failure by Infectious Causes*

Diseases and agents	Clinical signs	Comments and diagnosis aids
Parvoviral Infection Parvovirus	Vary with gestational stage at infection. Usually in gilts. Increases in returns to heat, failure to farrow, mummies, stillbirths, and neonatal mortality. Fewer pigs per litter. There seldom are abortions or fetal anomalies. The dams are normal.	A major cause of embryonic and fetal death, more often in gilts. Infection usually endemic and inapparent. Diagnosis by IFAT on lungs of mummies <16 cm long.
Porcine reproductive and respiratory syndrome (PRRS) Arterivirus	Sows may be sick from primary infection and abort, or abortions may occur several weeks after sow infected due to fetal infection. Decreased conception and farrowing rates. Increases in stillborns, weak pigs, mummies, premature farrowings and last trimester abortions. Improved reproductive performance after 3-5 months.	Respiratory signs and illness may be in any age group. PCR on serum from acutely ill sows or serology on convalescent sows; identify virus in fresh or fixed tissues of acutely affected neonates, or PCR on fluids from multiple aborted piglets.
Leptospirosis *Leptospira* spp.	Initial outbreak: Abortions and stillbirths common in late pregnancy. Piglets often weak and many die within a few days. Illness seldom noticed in dams.	After one failure, dams often breed successfully. Focal nephritis and hepatitis may be in fetuses or older swine. Diagnosis: by herd serology or by IFAT, PCR on fetal tissues.
Pseudorabies (PRV) Herpesvirus	Depends on gestational stage at infection; initially, abortions or respiratory signs. CNS signs or sudden deaths in young piglets; mortality often high, decreasing with age. Immune sows show no signs.	If endemic, reproductive signs less common than CNS or respiratory signs. Diagnosis by serology, virus isolation, IHC, PCR. Eradicated from the US since 2004.
Porcine circovirus type 2 (PCV2) Family Circoviridae	A common virus in swine population that may cause myoclonia congenita. It is associated with sporadic outbreaks of fetal death and/or mummification.	PCR may detect PCV2 in serum or tissues of presuckle piglets with myoclonia congenita. Lesions and virus detectable in hearts of aborted or mummified fetuses.
Brucellosis *Brucella suis*	Infertility common. Any manifestation of reproductive failure may occur. Abortions at any stage of pregnancy. In adults, lameness or paralysis. In older boars, orchitis.	Disease nearing eradication in the US. A serious zoonosis. Diagnosis by various serologic tests.

* Other less likely causes of reproductive failure include influenza, inclusion body rhinitis, classical swine fever, African swine fever, Japanese B encephalitis, and virulent enteroviral infections. Sporadic microbiologic causes include miscellaneous bacterial infections. Mycotoxins in feed are anecdotally reported but not proven. Any acute generalized illness during advanced pregnancy can lead to abortion.

Key: CNS-central nervous system; IFAT-immunofluorescent antibody test; IHC-immunohistochemistry; PCR-polymerase chain reaction

Respiratory Diseases*

Disease and etiologic agent	Clinical signs	Lesions gross-micro	Diagnostic aids, comments
Mycoplasmal pneumonia *Mycoplasma hyopneumoniae*	Persistent, dry cough, retarded growth, high morbidity/low mortality. Endemic in many herds.	Pneumonia and atelectasis in cranioventral lobules (gray-purple). Marked lymphoid hyperplasia around airways.	History and lesions are suggestive of diagnosis. FAT and IHC applied to lung tissue or PCR of airway swabs. Serology useful on a herd basis.
Atrophic rhinitis *Bordetella bronchiseptica* and/or toxigenic *Pasteurella multocida*	Sneezing, snorting, nasal discharge, epistaxis. Tear staining at medial canthi. Usually a deviation of snouts in a few pigs.	Variable turbinate atrophy. Perhaps deviation of snout. Tear staining. Secondary pneumonia often present.	Based on signs, history of reduced performance, typical lesions at necropsy or at slaughter. Culture and identify the agent(s) from turbinates or nasal swabs. Confirm toxigenicity.
Pneumonic pasteurellosis *Pasteurella multocida*	Coughing, dyspnea, fever, prostration.	Firm, fibrinous pneumonia cranioventrally and extending into diaphragmatic lobes. Variable pleuritis, perhaps adhesions/abscesses.	Culture *Pasteurella multocida* from lung lesions, possibly also from parenchymatous organs. Gray, firm, and subacute nature of lung lesions are suggestive of pasteurellosis. Organism a frequent, secondary, respiratory pathogen.
Inclusion body rhinitis Cytomegalovirus	Sneezing, nasal discharge in young piglets with variable mortality. Possibly dead, mummified or weak piglets at farrowing.	In young pigs: rhinitis with edema, petechial hemorrhages and a mucopurulent nasal exudate.	Large, almost pathognomonic, intranuclear inclusions in enlarged epithelial type cells (turbinates, Harderian and lachrymal glands, kidney, choroid plexus, other sites). Signs and lesion strongly suggest the diagnosis.
Pleuropneumonia (APP) *Actinobacillus pleuropneumoniae*	**Acute:** High temperatures, prostration, dyspnea, mouth breathing, perhaps bloody foam from nose. Short course, high morbidity and mortality. **Chronic:** chronic cough, unthriftiness	Pneumonia is firm, necrotic and bloody with fibrinous pleuritis. Chronic cases have pleural adhesions often with necrotic masses in lungs. Common in diaphragmatic lobes.	Signs and lesions are highly suggestive. Isolate agent from lung lesions and identify serotype. Serologically identify carrier herds by ELISA or CF tests.
Swine influenza (SIV) Influenza type A Subtypes H1N1 and H3N2 most common; diversity recognized.	Sudden onset, rapid spread of fever, serous nasal discharge, dyspnea, prostration. This is followed by loud coughing, and usually rapid recovery in seven days.	Multifocal to diffuse red firmness. Usually has lobular anteroventral distribution. Secondary bacterial pneumonia is common.	History and signs are very suggestive. Morbidity high, mortality low. Confirm presence of SIV by PCR or ELISA on nasal swabs or by PCR, IHC, FAT or VI from lung tissue. Serology by IHA or ELISA. Subtype determined by PCR.

Continued on next page

Respiratory Diseases* (continued)

Disease and etiologic agent	Clinical signs	Lesions gross-micro	Diagnostic aids, comments
Porcine reproductive and respiratory syndrome virus (PRRSV) Arterivirus	Respiratory disease and poor reproductive performance. High pre-weaning mortality. Respiratory dyspnea, fever and prolonged course, usually with abundant secondary agents.	In young pigs, focal or diffuse interstitial pneumonia in any or all lobes. Generally swollen lymph nodes. Perhaps secondary bronchopneumonia.	Chronic respiratory disease in growing swine. Identify virus in lung by IHC, FAT, or PCR. Isolate virus and identify. Demonstrate rising antibody titers in herd. Bronchoalveolar lavage is good specimen for PCR and isolation. Sequencing commonly performed by PCR.
Pseudorabies (PRV) Herpesvirus	Central nervous system (CNS) signs predominate in neonates and the very young. (Sudden death common in very young) Swine >3 weeks old: sneezing, coughing, nasal discharge, dyspnea	**Gross:** often no lesions. Perhaps rhinitis, tonsillitis, tracheitis, keratoconjunctivitis. **Histology:** Nonsuppurative meningoencephalitis. Necrotic bronchitis, bronchiolitis, alveolitis.	Isolate and identify virus. Histopath with IHC. FAT on tonsil, spleen, brain. Serologic tests reveal herd infection. PRV was eradicated from US commercial swine in 2004. PRV should now be thought of as a foreign disease and all suspicious cases reported and investigated.

* Parasitisms with respiratory signs include ascariasis (roundworm migration) and lungworm infection.

Key: CF-complement fixation; ELISA-enzyme-linked immunosorbent assay; FAT-fluorescent antibody test; HI-hemagglutination inhibition; IHA-indirect hemagglutination; IHC-immunohistochemistry; PCR-polymerase chain reaction; VI-virus isolation

Skin Lesions and Diseases

Name	Etiology	Signs-lesions	Comments
Actinobacillus suis infection	*Actinobacillus suis*	Unusual but in feeding/finishing and mature swine, the lesions are raised, red and rhomboid.	Signs, internal and cutaneous lesions can (rarely) resemble those of acute erysipelas
Aural hematoma	Trauma to ear followed by hemorrhage between skin and cartilage	Thickening and inflammation of ear over organizing hematoma. Lesions can be very large.	Trauma from many causes: bites, violent head shaking, commingling.
Dermatosis vegetans	Semi-lethal hereditary defect affecting occasional pigs.	Coronary band lesion on one or more feet of neonate, which leads to hoof deformity. Red macules expand, become papillomatous.	Defect originally in Landrace breed. Most affected piglets die within a few weeks. Many survivors have interstitial pneumonia.
Epitheliogenesis imperfecta	Congenital defect.	Missing areas of skin since birth, often over back or rump, perhaps mouth.	Small lesions often heal by scarring.
Erysipelas	*Erysipelothrix rhusiopathiae*	**Acute:** Raised, rhomboid lesions. **Chronic:** Peeling plaques often over back. Necrosis of parts of ears, tail.	Acute skin lesions often resolve if animal recovers promptly. Skin lesions appear slightly after acute febrile stage of disease.
Greasy pig disease	*Staphylococcus hyicus* skin infection	Brownish lesions in axilla and groin spread to head, face, other areas, perhaps mouth. Lesions dark, greasy, often extensive.	Triggering factors are poorly understood. Irritation of skin may precede the infection. Treatment seldom is satisfactory.
Necrotic ear syndrome	Trauma, vasculitis, often bites, and secondary infection.	Areas of ulceration, infection and necrosis in ear(s).	Infection occasionally results in septicemia and death.
Pediculosis (lice)	*Haematopinus suis* louse.	Rubbing, scratching, anemia. Eggs attached to hair on jowls, flanks, inner surface of legs, behind ears.	Leads to unthriftiness and anemia. Lice sometimes transmit pox virus.
Photodynamic dermatitis	Photodynamic agents (plants or drugs) plus sunlight.	White areas of skin inflamed and pruritic. Severe peeling of areas of necrotic skin.	Many plants and drugs are photodynamic. Conjunctivitis often accompanies the dermatitis.
Pityriasis rosea	Unknown but some evidence of hereditary predisposition.	Raised, expanding circular lesions in 12-14 week old pigs. Lesions usually on ventral abdomen, less often elsewhere.	Lesions resolve within a few weeks without treatment. Disease may go unnoticed unless ventrum is examined.
Porcine dermatopathy and nephropathy syndrome (PDNS)	Mechanism unknown but associated with post-viral (PCV2, PRRSV, CSF)* infection, perhaps an immune mediated disease.	Red to purple, circular 1 cm lesions appear on perineal, ham, ventral regions that may enlarge and coalesce. Nephropathy also present may lead to death in days to weeks.	Diagnosis by recognition and histopathology on skin and kidney. Usually sporadic but morbidity can approach 10%. No treatment.

Continued on next page

Skin Lesions and Diseases (continued)

Name	Etiology	Signs-lesions	Comments
Pox	Swine pox virus	Initial 1-2 cm round to oval lesions on ventrum but can extend over the body. Papule, vesicle, pustule and scab stages.	All age groups susceptible. Usually seen in young, growing pigs. Pox virus sometimes transmitted by lice. Congenital pox occurs sporadically.
Pustular dermatitis	Lancefield type C *Streptococci*	Pustules on posterioventral abdomen, inguinal area, inner thighs, perhaps eyes, lips, ears. Pustules rupture, are replaced by black scabs.	Most pigs recover in a few weeks. Provide clean bedding, improve sanitation. Recovery perhaps hastened by antibiotics in water or feed.
Ringworm	Usually *Microsporum nanum* or *Trichophyton verrucosum.*	Roughly circular, expanding hairless areas that develop crested scabs. Non-pruritic.	Usually self-limiting. Contagious to humans. Occasionally caused by other fungi. Usually seen in old swine and quite common in sows.
Skin necrosis of piglets	Skin abrasion with secondary infection.	Abrasive lesions on knees, fetlocks, coronets, hocks, or elbows lead to septicemia; often high mortality.	Lesions often are more serious than realized. Less abrasive surfaces or adequate bedding are necessities.
Sunburn	Excessive sunshine on skin	Pigs may "drop to belly" from pain on sunburned back. Reddening, thickening, peeling of most exposed skin, usually on back and ears. Unpigmented skin more susceptible.	If shade is provided, pigs will not lay in the sun.
Vesiculating viral diseases	Foot-and-mouth disease (FMD), Vesicular stomatitis (VS), Vesicular exanthema (VE).	Round to oval vesicles on feet, in and around the mouth, on snout, in nostrils, occasionally elsewhere.	Lesions similar in all vesiculating viral diseases and cannot be used to differentiate. Report all promptly!
Vices	Tail or flank biting; savaging of moribund swine.	Tail or flank bite wounds. Moribund swine often have red, linear bite marks.	Overcrowding and idleness are thought to contribute to development of vices.

* Key: PCV2-porcine circovirus type 2; PRRSV-porcine reproductive and respiratory syndrome virus; CSF-classical swine fever

Vesiculating Viral Diseases

Disease	Family-genus of virus	Other animals affected	Comments
Foot-and-mouth disease (FMD)	Picornaviridae *Aphthovirus*	Most ruminants, wild and domestic. Several lab and wild animals.	US free of FMD. Eradicated nine times from US.
Vesicular stomatitis (VS)	Rhabdoviridae *Vesiculovirus*	Cattle, horses, certain wildlife, humans	Endemic in Carolinas, Georgia. Periodic epidemics in many other states.
Vesicular exanthema (VE) San Miguel sea lion virus (SMSLV)	Caliciviridae *Calicivirus*	Swine, sea lions, opal eye fish, several kinds of seals and other marine animals.	No VE since 1956. SMSLV in marine animals off coast of California may be a threat to swine.
Swine vesicular disease	Picornaviridae *Enterovirus*	Swine; occasionally humans	Never in US. Last outbreak in Italy, 1995.

Section IX

Appendix A

Abbreviations and Acronyms

Infectious diseases

AR: atrophic rhinitis

APP: *Actinobacillus pleuropneumoniae*

ASF: African swine fever

BVD: bovine viral diarrhea

EMC: encephalomyocarditis

FMD: foot and mouth disease

HC: hog cholera

HPS: *Haemophilus parasuis*

PCMV: porcine cytomegalovirus

PMWS: postweaning multisystemic wasting syndrome

PCV: porcine circovirus

PED: porcine epidemic diarrhea

PPE: porcine proliferative enteropathy

PPV: porcine parvovirus

PRDC: porcine respiratory disease complex

PRRS: porcine reproductive and respiratory syndrome

PRV: pseudorabies virus

SD: swine dysentery

SIV: swine influenza

SMSLV: San Miguel sea lion viral disease

SMEDI: stillbirth, mummified fetuses, embryonic death, infertility

TGE: transmissible gastroenteritis

VE: vesicular exanthema

VS: vesicular stomatitis

Non-infectious diseases

OA: osteoarthritis

OCD: osteochondrosis

PHS: porcine hypogalactia syndrome

PSS: porcine stress syndrome

Nutrition

ADG: average daily gain

ADFI: average daily feed intake

FE: feed efficiency

Laboratory terms

AI: artificial insemination

CF: complement fixation

CPE: cytopathic effect

ELISA: enzyme-linked immunosorbent assay

EM: electron microscopy

EPG: eggs per gram

ET: embryo transfer

FA: fluorescent antibody

HA: hemagglutination

HI: hemagglutination inhibition

IF: immunofluorescence

IHA: indirect hemagglutination

IHC: immunohistochemistry

PCR: polymerase chain reaction

SN: serum neutralization

VI: virus isolation

VN: virus neutralization

Organizations

AASV: American Association of Swine Veterinarians

AAVLD: American Association of Veterinary Laboratory Diagnosticians

Organizations (continued)

AHI: Animal Health Institute

APHIS: Animal and Plant Health Inspection Service

VS: Veterinary Services

CVM: Center for Veterinary Medicine

FADDL: Foreign Animal Disease Diagnostic Laboratory

FSIS: Food Safety Inspection Service

NADC: National Animal Disease Center

NIAA: National Institute for Animal Agriculture

NPB: National Pork Board

NPPC: National Pork Producers Council

NRC: National Research Council

NRCS: Natural Resources Conservation Service

USAHA: US Animal Health Association

VFDC: Veterinary Feed Directive Coalition

Documents-publications

ADAA: Animal Drug Availability Act

GATT: General Agreement on Tariffs and Trade

NAFTA: North American Free Trade Agreement

JSHAP: *Journal of Swine Health and Production* (AASV journal)

SHPA: Swine Health Protection Act

SHER: Swine Health and Epidemiology Report

VFD: Veterinary Feed Directive

Food Safety

AMDUCA: Animal Medicinal Drug Use Clarification Act

EQIP: Environmental Quality Incentive Program

FSIS: Food Safety Inspection Service

HACCP: Hazard Analysis Critical Control Points

PQA: Pork Quality Assurance

Swine Industry Terminology

Following are some terms used in the swine-raising industry. Although many of the terms have never been defined precisely, the definitions give some idea as to their meaning:

Acclimatization

A period of time for new breeding stock to become immune to disease organisms on the farm. This is usually by isolation of these animals from the herd but intentional exposure to potential pathogens on the recipient farm such as commingling with culls. The goal is for incoming breeding stock to become immune to and cease shedding of those agents. Acclimatization is often performed at the same time as the period of isolation.

Isolation

Animals that have a risk of introducing or carrying disease are placed in a location isolated from the herd. Incoming breeding stock frequently are housed at an isolated site, observed, and tested for disease exposure. Often, isolation and acclimatization are simultaneous.

All-in/all-out system (AIAO)

A production method where all pigs in a group are placed in a facility, there are no additions to the group following placement, and all are removed before any other pigs are placed. Usually, pigs are born in as short (one to two weeks) a period as possible, started, raised and sold together. Each subsequent group is separated physically and has separate air space. No pigs are added to the group at any time. The facilities are totally depopulated, cleaned and disinfected as each group exits. There are many disease control advantages. There is only one age group of pigs in the location.

Continuous production system

Any rearing system under which the pigs use facilities continuously or nearly so or where a facility is not completely depopulated before more pigs are added. Often the pigs are not started, raised, or sold together which is the opposite of the all-in/all-out system. Pigs may be added to groups to make maximum use of facilities. These systems have groups of pigs of different ages in the same location.

Conventional (farrow-to-finish) system

A swine production system where all stages of production (breeding, gestation, farrowing, nursery, and finishing) are on the same site, often housed together or in immediately adjacent buildings. The building(s) may be subdivided or partitioned into sections for each stage of production.

Three-site production system

A system of raising pigs at three well-separated facilities. At site one there is breeding, gestation and farrowing. At site two there is a nursery. At site three there is a grower/finisher facility. All sites are run on an all-in/all-out basis. Some operators prefer to combine sites two and three and the operation may be referred to as a two-site system.

Isowean

The Isowean system is sometimes referred to as segregated rearing and may include a medication program known as medicated early weaning (MEW) or modified, medicated, early weaning (MMEW). Many features of medicated early weaning (below) are incorporated but pigs are weaned later than a specified age (e.g. 17 days of age). Weaning age and medication depend on disease(s) in the source herd to be controlled by early weaning and medication.

Medicated early weaning (MEW)

A system of raising pigs under which piglets are weaned at four to five days of age and medicated continuously from birth until they are 10-20 days old. The piglets are then raised in an isolated nursery until they are five to eight weeks old and moved through the system as a group in all-in/all-out production. The dams are medicated from about five days prior to farrowing to the time their piglets are selected and removed. The system is used to reduce or eliminate pathogens that might be transmitted to piglets from the dams.

Nucleus herd

A nucleus herd is a highly selected herd of swine containing the best breeding stock obtainable and from which selected animals will go to multiplier herds. Multiplier herds increase parent stock to be delivered to commercial farms and swine producers for production.

Specific pathogen free (SPF) system

A method of obtaining surgically derived piglets and raising them artificially or on foster sows believed to be free of specific diseases. The system prevents the pigs from being infected from their dam since, with a few exceptions, piglets are biologically sterile prior to birth. Piglets usually are monitored for specific pathogens. The genetic background of the piglets is maintained. Primary SPF pigs are surgically derived and are raised away from contact with conventional pigs. Secondary SPF pigs are those raised from primary SPF pigs. They are farrowed naturally and reared conventionally.

Index

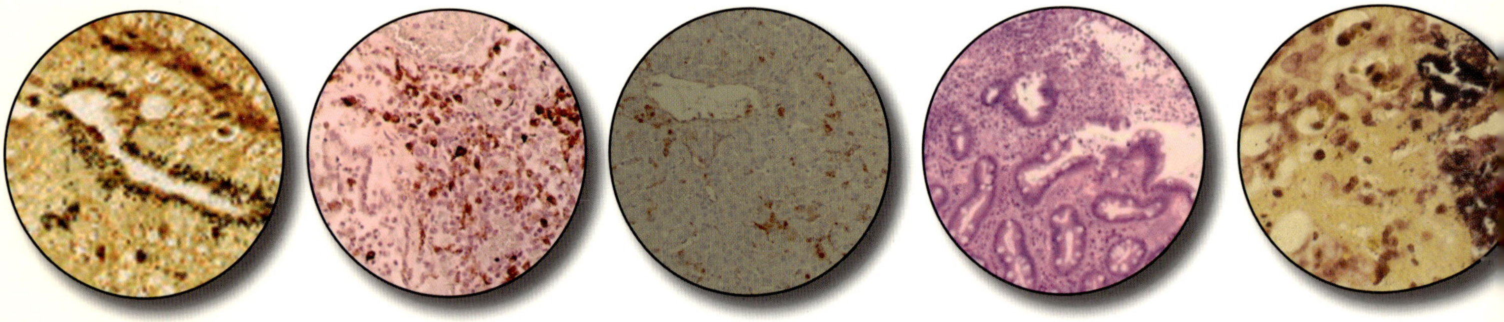

Published by the American Association of Swine Veterinarians
ISBN 978-0-9843503-0-8